L.J.FLANDERS

CELL
WORKOUT

First published in Great Britain in 2015 by LC Books

First published in 2016 by Hodder & Stoughton

An Hachette UK company

A CIP catalogue record for this title is available from the British Library

Trade Paperback ISBN 978 1 473 65601 7
eBook ISBN 978 1 473 65602 4

Typeset in Univers by Beachstone
beachstone.co.uk

Printed and bound in by Firmengruppe APPL, aprinta druck, Wemding, Germany

Hodder & Stoughton policy is to use papers that are natural, renewable and recyclable products and made from wood grown in sustainable forests. The logging and manufacturing processes are expected to conform to the environmental regulations of the country of origin.

Hodder & Stoughton Ltd
Carmelite House
50 Victoria Embankment
London EC4Y 0DZ

www.hodder.co.uk

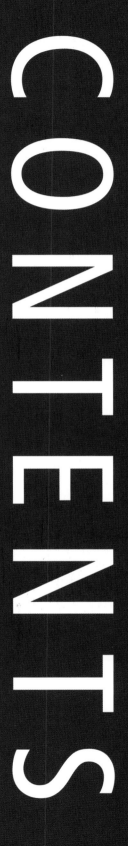

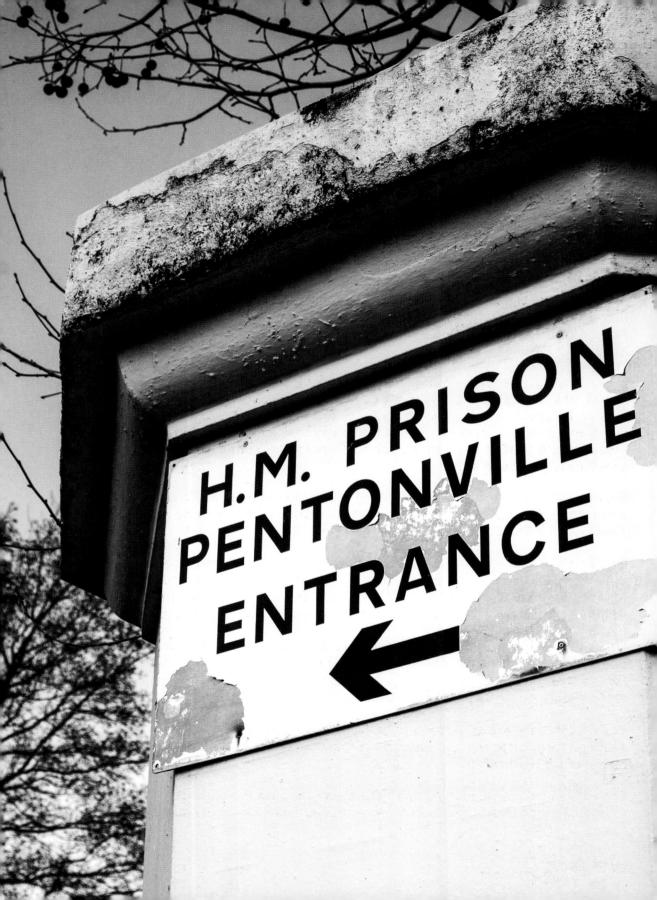

WHY I WROTE THIS BOOK ...

In prison, people can discover new things and improve themselves in many ways; faith, fitness, a new language, education, skills and qualifications that may lead to job opportunities. In my case, I decided to make use of my time and channelled my energy into exercise and fitness.

So what motivated me to write this book? Firstly, to satisfy my own craving to keep fit. With limited access to the gym, I began working out in my cell. But there are only so many standard press ups or sit ups a person can do without getting bored or hitting a plateau.

During my time in Pentonville I studied to become a personal trainer and once qualified I got a job in the prison gym. It wasn't long before inmates, even my friends who were writing in to me, were asking me to write them a 'cell workout'. At that time, I didn't have the expertise or knowledge to provide what they were looking for.

Like many people who are interested in their personal fitness, I only knew the basics of training, using weights and cardio. After scouring the prison library looking for sources to help write these programs, I soon realised that information was very limited, barely skimming the surface of what I was looking for. In fact I was unable to find any other book that contained suitable exercises designed specifically for use in a cell.

Eventually I put pen to paper, thinking of various exercises for each body part, writing the descriptions and drawing the diagrams. This lengthy process would eventually become the blueprint for this book.

On my release I then had access to the Internet and spent many hours researching the overwhelming volume of information. Months later I finally had a clear vision of what I wanted my book to be – a definitive and extensive guide to bodyweight training. That is exactly what I had wanted but couldn't find, when I needed it most.

Upon leaving prison, being able to focus on this book has helped me in every possible way. With no experience of writing or self publishing a book, I admit that I was naïve. I definitely did not fully appreciate the challenges that I would face, let alone the five months of training it took to get ready for the photographs.

But after three years of hard work, determination and a lot of help from my friends, seeing it through to the end gives me a massive sense of achievement and makes all the effort worthwhile.

From my initial vision, to making it a reality, this book is the outcome of my personal journey through prison and after. I hope in some way it can help you on yours.

WHAT IS A CELL WORKOUT?

This is a term often used quite loosely, without much meaning or understanding. To me and the basis of the content of this book – the 'Cell Workout' uses the bodyweight resistance training method and can be performed in a confined space: 6 by 8 is more than enough; and it doesn't have to be a prison cell. The training goal is simple – total physical fitness combined with a positive state of mind.

Bodyweight training is the oldest form of exercise, requiring no weights or equipment. This method has recently shown a big resurgence in popularity. It forms the basis for almost every type of exercise – Pilates, yoga, calisthenics, plyometrics, gymnastics and most sports. Using this purest and most basic form of exercise can tone, sculpt and build your body.

This training method will improve all aspects of physical fitness. It is made up of many components: health (strength, muscular and cardiovascular endurance, flexibility and body composition) and skill-related fitness (speed, power, reaction time, co-ordination, balance and agility).

As human beings we need a balance between them all; it's no good concentrating on one component while neglecting another. It's not just the aesthetics that count – you also need to be healthy inside. Cardiovascular exercise is good for bone density, blood circulation, the respiratory system and internal organs. Your heart is the most important muscle of all and exercising will make it stronger.

So what do you really want to achieve? This book will educate and inform, guiding you through the process of understanding your training goals and how to make bodyweight training work for you. Whatever your personal goal may be, there are exercises suitable for any age, ability or fitness level.

Many people who exercise, don't have the expertise to realise the potential of their own body. Work through the chapters and learn how to achieve the results you want. There are explanations of the components of physical (health and skill-related) fitness; how certain training principles and methods are applied; training terminology and various guidelines for resistance, cardio and flexibility training.

The majority of the book is made up of an extensive range of exercises, divided into muscle groups. The opening of each chapter explains the basic function, movement and purpose of the muscles. This is followed by the exercises, giving the primary and secondary muscle groups being used; a step-by-step description and photos showing how to perform the exercise.

The final section of the book outlines my own interpretation of the 'Cell Workout'. A 10 week workout for beginner, intermediate and advanced fitness levels, with rep ranges, set duration, number of sets, rest breaks and different intensities.

The first 6 weeks are bodyweight workouts that will improve your muscular strength and endurance. Performing the exercises with control and precision is the most important starting point. The exercises show a natural progression and further divides the muscles groups every 2 weeks. This is followed by 4 weeks of cardio workouts, for cardiovascular endurance, speed and power. All the individual workouts include a warm up and cool down to promote flexibility.

Following the 10 week cell workout will torch body fat and significantly change your body composition, therefore improving in all components of health and skill-related fitness.

The workouts can be adapted to suit your needs, as there is no such thing as a generic workout. How you want to look and feel is unique to you. As your ability and knowledge improves, you will simply rework, re-energise and progress.

Exercising is also beneficial for your emotional well-being. It produces a natural high which has a positive effect on our physical and mental state. Exercising will lift your spirits, and leave you feeling more positive and energised. The relaxation and meditation chapters give information on how to calm and focus the mind.

My main aim is to motivate you to begin an exercise regime that will become part of your everyday life. Circumstances or situations that we cannot change for whatever reason shouldn't stop us achieving. Even during times of adversity, we still need to strive to be physically and mentally strong.

You already have the vital tools to keep fit – your own body. The possibilities are limitless, you will always be improving and perfecting to achieve your personal best.

Get the body you want – **Inside & Out.**

THE BENEFITS OF BODYWEIGHT TRAINING

Bodyweight training is a form of exercise where the weight of your own body provides the resistance for the exercise.

The physical benefits of bodyweight training include: increased fitness levels and strength, builds muscle and tones the body, improves bone density, boosts cardiovascular fitness, burns fat, helps maintain a healthy weight or weight loss, promotes flexibility and balance, will improve how your body moves in a functional manner.

Like other forms of exercise, bodyweight training has the following health benefits: reduces risk of major illnesses, joint problems and injury, boosts energy levels, promotes better sleep quality and can have a positive effect on mental health.

The fact that the only weight being used is that of your own body shouldn't be viewed as a disadvantage. Even the simplest bodyweight exercise can be easily modified to challenge any fitness level and can be progressed or regressed to meet your individual needs, reducing the risk of injury.

There are many ways that you can progress:

Perfect form: quality rather than quantity.
Volume: increase the number of reps and sets.
Intensity: how hard you train, how long you train and length of rest period.
Tempo: fast, slow or explosive.
ROM: increase full range of movement.
Leverage: decreased angle of body position.
Symmetric: parallel hand or feet placement.
Asymmetric: staggered hand or feet placement.
Unilateral: single limb exercise.
Difficulty: work towards a more advanced variation.
Equipment: pull up and dip bar, gymnastic rings, rope, weighted vest, suspension trainer, plyo box, wobble board.

Bodyweight training can be performed alongside other forms of resistance training. Additional specific bodyweight training equipment can be used if available, but all the exercises in this book can be performed without.

Without weights you can still achieve any training goal. Your muscles will respond to tension, whether it's a barbell, machine or your own bodyweight. If challenged to a high enough stimulus, they will react and adapt, resulting in a complete and balanced workout.

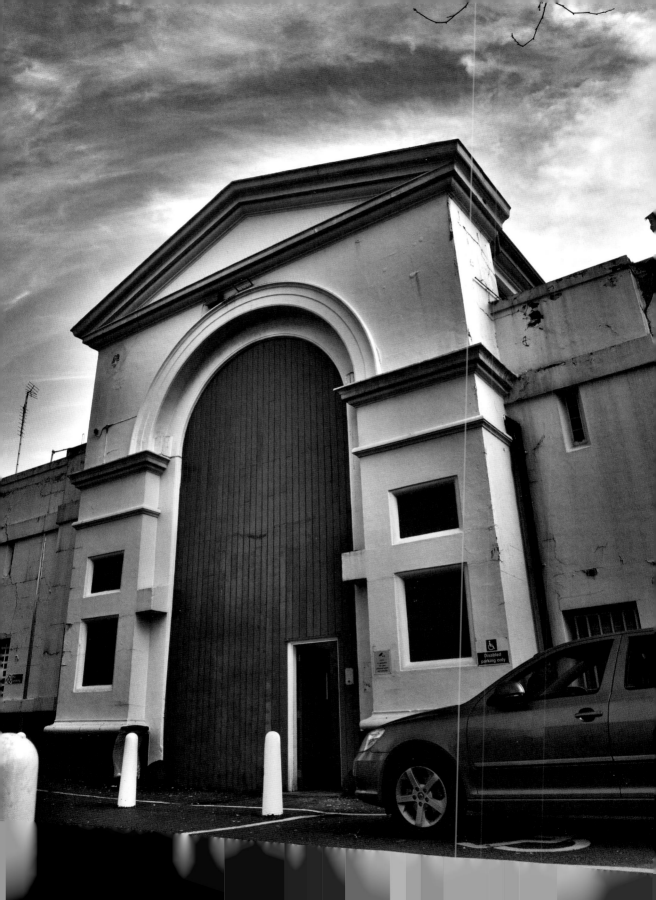

ANATOMICAL POSITION

FRONT (ANTERIOR)

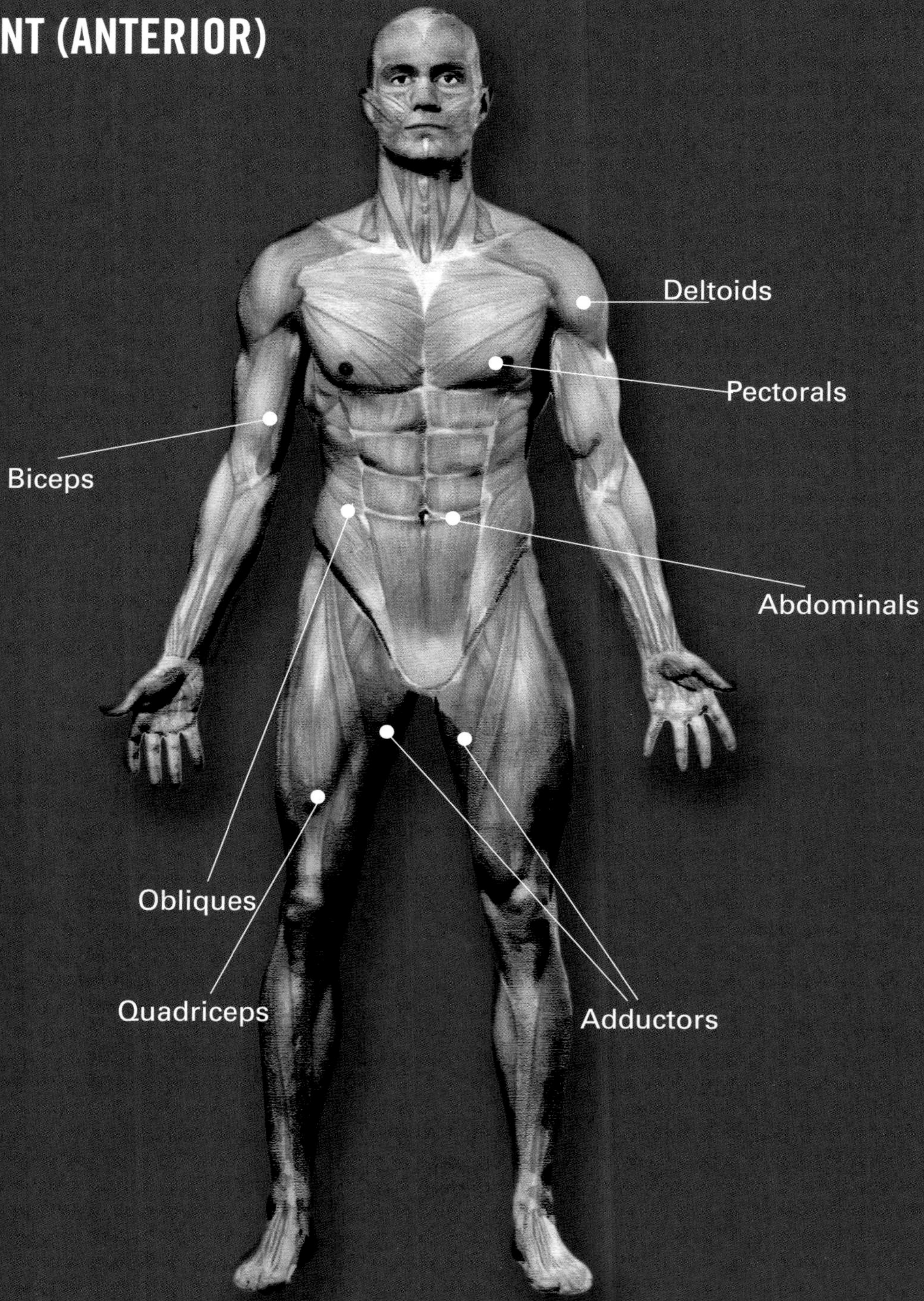

Deltoids

Pectorals

Biceps

Abdominals

Obliques

Quadriceps

Adductors

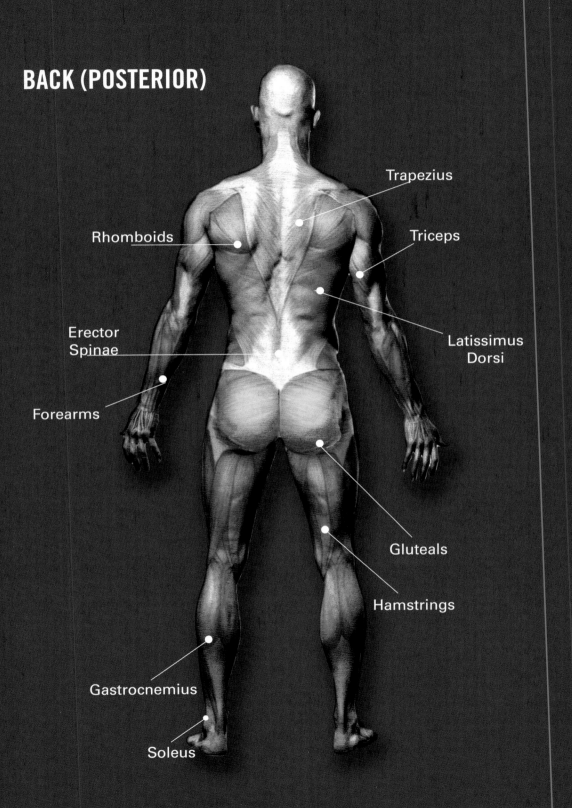

BACK (POSTERIOR)

Trapezius

Rhomboids

Triceps

Erector
Spinae

Latissimus
Dorsi

Forearms

Gluteals

Hamstrings

Gastrocnemius

Soleus

BASIC TRAINING PRINCIPLES: FITT

Frequency is how often you exercise. You will want to put your body under enough stress to adapt and also allow enough time for healing and adaption to occur without over training.

Intensity is how hard and how much effort you put into your training.

For **resistance training**, your workload is the way to measure your intensity. In weight lifting terms the percentage of one-rep max (1RM) is the method of monitoring intensity and progression. With bodyweight training you cannot alter the amount of resistance. The three components are: i) number of repetitions ii) time it takes to complete all repetitions in a set or whole training session iii) how hard you work.

For **cardiovascular training**, Heart Rate (HR) and Rating of Perceived Exertion (RPE) is the way to measure your intensity.

Resting Heart Rate (RHR) is measured in beats per minute (bpm) and can indicate your level of fitness when taken before any sort of exercise, preferably in the morning. Your RHR can be monitored and measured by taking your pulse at the wrist or from the side of your neck, using your index and middle fingers while you are sitting down. Then count the number of beats in 60 seconds (bpm).

Maximum Heart Rate (MHR) average is measured as: 220 – age (years) = MHR. From this measurement you can then set yourself a target heart rate.

Target Heart Rate (THR) is selecting the percentage of the MHR you want to work at. So if your MHR is 180bpm and you want to work at a THR of 50%, you multiply 180bpm by 50%, which gives you a recommended THR zone of 90bpm.

To monitor your heart rate during exercise, you will need to periodically take your pulse to measure your bpm.

Rating of Perceived Exertion (RPE) is a rating of your physical exertion during exercise. The scale starts at 6 (no exertion at all) to 20 (maximum exertion). To rate yourself, you need to take into account the physical stress, effort and fatigue of working muscles and level of breathing.

Type is the method of training you use to improve the component of fitness you have chosen.

Time is how long you spend training. This depends on the type of training you have chosen. The level of intensity you work at will also determine how long you train for.

MAIN TRAINING PRINCIPLES

Specificity is when planning your training program, the goals you set need to be specific to what you are trying to achieve and the component of fitness you want to improve in. The changes that your muscles, organs or systems go through will depend on the type of training you choose.

Individuality is the fact that everyone is different, with varying abilities and response to training.

Progression is to improve in your training program and over time, progress on to harder exercises and movements. With bodyweight training, the resistance used is your bodyweight. Progression is achieved by increased reps, sets, decreased rest breaks, different tempos and moving on to more advanced exercises.

Overload is for your body to develop (muscle, organs or systems). Your training needs to be demanding and challenging enough to bring on adaption. When working harder, muscles will get stronger. This principle works alongside progression.

Adaptation will occur after long-term training. Your body will adapt to the type of training you undertake, resulting in improved efficiency, less effort and less muscle breakdown. This is why you need variety and increase the stimulus to work harder and again react to a greater demand. Adaptation occurs at different times for each individual.

Recovery process happens after each workout, no matter what training program you choose. After activity you need to rest your body in order for it to repair and recover. The adaptation your body goes through happens after you have finished your workout, not during. Without recovery you are more likely to sustain an injury and your progression will reduce. The harder you train, the longer you need to rest.

Variation should be included, as using different training methods will prevent boredom from the same type of training, without diverting from your training goal. Variety using the same targeted muscle group can be a good change.

Reversibility is when you stop or reduce training levels to a point where adaption doesn't occur. This will reverse your ability to efficiently perform certain exercises. Maintenance programmes are a good way to reduce the loss of progress – use it or lose it!

SOME TRAINING TERMINOLOGY

Exercise is a movement designed to challenge and develop the body.

Breathing during an exercise; the simplest form is to breathe in during the eccentric 'lowering' phase and breathe out during the concentric 'lifting' phase.

Technique is the way in which an exercise is performed, a combination of many factors.

Form is performing a movement specific to that exact exercise, using safety to maximise results. Using good form will reduce the risk of injury.

Muscle contraction is a process in which tension is developed within muscle tissue. During muscle contraction the tension may cause the muscle to stay the same length, lengthen or shorten.

Roles of Muscles, working together to produce different bodily movements and their roles may change depending on the movement.

Agonist 'primary' muscles are directly involved in producing and controlling movement.

Antagonist is the opposing muscle to the working agonist muscle. When the agonist muscle contracts causing a movement to occur, the antagonist would typically relax so as to not impede the agonist. The role of the antagonist muscle is also to control, slow down or stop a movement.

Synergist 'secondary' muscles stabilise a joint around which a movement is occuring. They assist the agonist 'primary' muscles to function correctly as well as helping to perform the movement.

Fixator muscles help stabilise and eliminate unwanted movement of the origin of the agonist and help it function efficiently.

Types of Exercise

Compound exercises are multi-joint exercises using more than one muscle group at the same time. With one large muscle group being worked primarily and smaller muscle groups recruited secondarily.

Isolation exercises use only one muscle group or joint at a time.

Types of Movement and Contraction

Isometric contraction happens when a muscle is under tension, but is not changing length and there is little or no movement occurring.

Isotonic contraction happens when tension develops to a point and then remains constant while the muscle changes length to create a movement.

Concentric contraction happens when the working muscle shortens. This is also referred to as the 'positive' lifting phase of the exercise.

Eccentric contraction happens when the working muscle lengthens. This is also referred to as the 'negative' lowering phase of the exercise.

Range Of Movement (ROM) is the movement from full flexion to full extension.

Rep or repetition is a complete motion of an exercise.

Set is the specific number of reps performed before rest.

Rest break is the amount of time spent resting between each set.

Tempo is how fast each rep is performed, including both the concentric and eccentric phase. The most common tempo is 3-0-1-0. In an isometric exercise it is how long a position is held without moving for 30-60 seconds.

Volume is measured by how many exercises, reps and sets are completed during a workout.

Overtraining is when the body is put under too much stress and is not then able to recover fully.

Delayed Onset Muscle Soreness (DOMS) is the pain and stiffness in trained muscles, felt most strongly 24 to 72 hours after strenuous exercise.

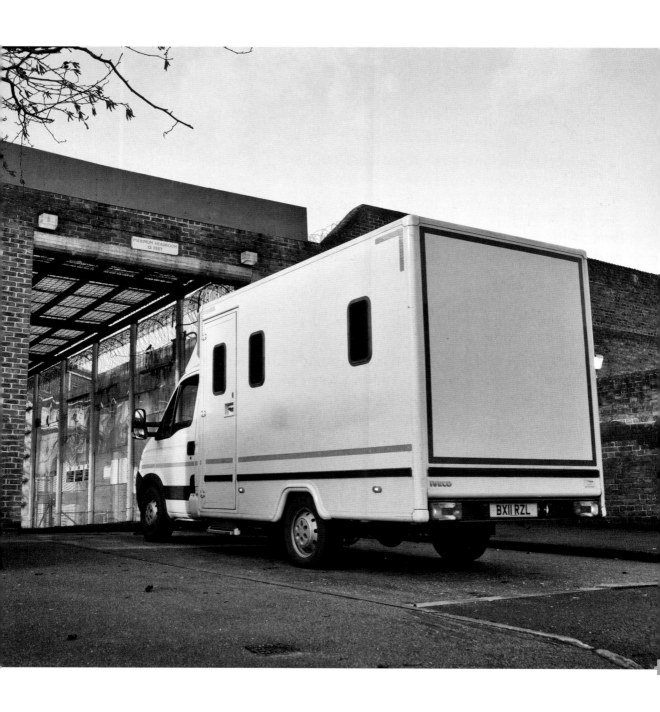

COMPONENTS OF TOTAL FITNESS

Fitness is a general term and can mean different things. It could be training for a specific sport or to improve in performing everyday tasks with ease.

The five components of total fitness:

Physical (health and skill).
Mental and emotional.
Medical.
Nutritional.
Social.

This book focuses mainly on health and skill-related fitness, which is achieved through physical exercise. Physical fitness is a state of general well-being. The level of difficulty to which each individual can perform an exercise will depend on various factors: age, gender, body type, diet, activity level, physical disabilities, illness, drugs, stress and environment.

COMPONENTS OF PHYSICAL FITNESS

Before designing your workout, it is important to understand the components of physical fitness. This will help establish more clearly your own objectives and make your exercise program more effective.

THE FIVE COMPONENTS OF HEALTH-RELATED FITNESS

Strength is the extent to which muscles can exert force by contracting against resistance. Strength training using bodyweight is mainly based on how hard the exercises are to perform, by you personally, with maximum effort, with the rep range being from 1-5 reps.

Muscular endurance is the muscular system's ability to work efficiently when performing for a sustained amount of time, (12+ reps with light to moderate resistance). With bodyweight training, as the resistance cannot be altered, how much you weigh and how conditioned you are can play a big part.

Cardiovascular endurance is the ability of the lungs and heart to intake and deliver oxygenated blood to working muscles and their ability to use it during continued aerobic training. Walking, jogging and running are the simplest ways of improving your cardiovascular system.

Flexibility is the ability to achieve an extended range of movement in a joint or group of joints without being impeded by excess tissue such as body fat or muscle mass. Flexibility can be improved with stretching exercises.

Body composition is the percentages of fat, bone and muscle in the human body. Body fat percentage is a good way to determine your health in addition to body weight. Fat and muscle weigh exactly the same, though muscle takes up less space on the body, which can really alter the way you look. A healthy male should be 13-17 percent fat. A healthy woman should be 20-25 percent fat.

An individual's body type will have an impact on their ability to perform basic daily tasks and actual physical exercise. There are three distinct body types:

Ectomorphs are naturally thin, with little body fat or muscle mass and find it difficult to gain weight (either muscle or fat).

Mesomorphs tend to be naturally lean, muscular and athletic.

Endomorphs are naturally prone to high fat storage and have trouble losing weight. Muscle mass may not be visible due to fat storage.

THE SIX COMPONENTS OF SKILL-RELATED FITNESS

Speed is the quickness of movement of a body part or parts and can be expressed as any one of, or combination of, the following: maximum speed, elastic strength (power) and speed endurance.

Power is the ability to exert maximum muscular contraction instantly in an explosive burst of movement. The two components of power are strength and speed.

Reaction time is the time between a stimulus and the time it takes for a muscular response.

Co-ordination is the ability to perform a movement using one or more body parts in a smooth, controlled and efficient way.

Balance is the ability to control the body's position, either while stationary or moving using the body's sensory functions.

Agility is the ability to quickly perform movements, changing the direction of the body in opposing directions efficiently and effectively.

RESISTANCE TRAINING

MUSCULAR STRENGTH

This component involves fully exhausting individual muscle groups during a workout. When selecting the exercises, they need to be challenging enough to work that muscle group to its maximum. An exercise becomes a strength exercise when the individual can perform no more than 1-5 intense reps with maximum effort and perfect form.

If the exercise is too easy and you can perform 5+ reps, then this becomes a muscular endurance exercise. The 1-Day Split: Full Body Split workout isn't recommended here as it doesn't allow each muscle group to be worked to its maximum within the 30-45 minutes.

The recommended splits are 2-Day Split: Upper Body and Lower Body Split or 3-Day Split: Push, Pull and Legs Split.

MUSCULAR SPEED AND POWER

This component is designed to increase muscular speed, power and explosiveness. The movements increase the strength and elasticity of muscle tissue to increase the speed and force of muscular contraction.

Cardio exercises are performed repetitively and rhythmically. Plyometric exercises involve the muscles rapidly going through a quick eccentric 'lengthening' phase to a powerful concentric 'shortening' phase. Plyometric exercises have a higher intensity than the cardio exercises. When selecting exercises from the cardio chapter, plyometric exercises are referred to as 'Plyo' in this book. There are additional plyometric exercises at the end of the chest chapter.

The 1-Day Split: Full Body Split is recommended, as you will be mainly training legs throughout the workout.

MUSCULAR ENDURANCE

This component allows your muscles to work continuously for a long duration without tiring. You should select exercises that you can perform 12+ reps without loss of form.

Circuit training is a good method for improving muscular endurance. It is set up using a number of different exercises being performed at different stations, for the specific time interval or rep count. This can also have some aerobic increasing effects. The difficulty level can be altered in various ways: time spent on each exercise, duration of rest period, number of exercises and circuits.

Any of the splits are suitable. 1-Day Split: Full Body Split is recommend as a good way to structure your workout.

RESISTANCE TRAINING GUIDELINES

Variables	Muscular Strength	Muscular Speed and Power	Muscular Endurance
Intensity	High	Vigorous	Moderate
Reps	1-5	5-10	12+
Rest between sets (minutes)	3-5	2-3	1-2
Sets per exercise	2-5	2-5	2-5
Duration (minutes)	30-45	30-45	30-45
Frequency (per week)	4-5	3-4	4-5
Method	2-Day or 3-Day Split	1-Day Split	Any Split

PROGRAM DESIGN

For resistance training, you will need to be specific with the exercises selected and the order of the exercises performed. This will have a big impact on the results of the workout. Use these guidelines on exercise selection to help plan your workout and make them more effective.

Muscular balance: with resistance training you need to work all of the major muscle groups so that the body progresses as a whole rather than isolated muscles being over worked.

Train large muscles first: depending on how many muscle groups are being trained during the workout, the largest muscle groups (agonist) should be trained first. The movements used to train these muscles will require the most energy to perform effectively.

Perform compound exercises first: perform the hardest compound exercises at the beginning of the workout as they require more skill, energy, co-ordination and use multi-joints. Then they will be performed safely, effectively and with good form, before fatigue sets in.

Train synergists and fixators last: if synergist 'secondary' muscles are trained prior to the agonist 'primary' muscles in a workout, they would fatigue quicker and not fulfill their role when it comes to helping the agonist muscles. This would mean that the larger muscle groups would then not be trained to their maximum potential.

Fixators contract to stabilise the body to provide the agonist with a solid base to work from. The core takes on the role of fixator in the majority of compound and multi-joint exercises. If trained prior to compound exercises and fatigue sets in, then they would not protect and align the spine during exercise.

TRAINING METHODS

SPLIT SYSTEM RESISTANCE TRAINING

The split system training method alternates major muscle groups by dividing them into separate workouts on different days throughout the week, with appropriate rest days. The split you chose will depend on the component you are trying to improve in. The basic split is 1-Day Split: Full Body Split which progresses to 2-Day Split: Upper Body and Lower Body Split and then the 3-Day Split: Push, Pull and Legs Split.

Scheduling your workouts – it is best to plan the week as Monday to Sunday, so that you know what muscle groups you are training on what day.

Depending on how many muscle groups you train per workout will determine the rest days. The fewer muscle groups in the workout means that the targeted muscles are worked to a higher intensity in the allotted time.

Different muscle groups require different recovery times, so your rest time will depend on the muscle group or groups you are training and the split being performed. See the guidelines that follow for more information. The recommended days off can be altered if you are still feeling sore or unusually tired and therefore not fully recovered.

1-DAY SPLIT: FULL BODY SPLIT

This split involves training the whole body in one workout, usually alternating days as one day on, one day off. With a training session lasting no longer than 30-45 minutes and lots of muscles groups being worked, there will not be enough time to perform a high number of sets or lots of exercises per muscle group.

This split is mainly used for the components of muscular endurance and muscular speed and power. A benefit of this split is that the muscle groups are worked regularly with one rest day in between.

2-DAY SPLIT: UPPER BODY AND LOWER BODY SPLIT

This split progresses and starts to divide the muscle groups and will take two days to train the entire body. With the upper body and lower body split, the first day you will train muscles in your upper body and the next day, the muscles in your lower body and abdominals.

Training the legs can be very demanding. Focusing solely on the lower body means the legs can be trained for longer and at a higher intensity. At the same time the upper body is resting and vice versa, followed by a rest day.

3-DAY SPLIT: PUSH, PULL AND LEGS SPLIT

This split is a further progression, splitting the muscle groups, taking three days to train the entire body. The theory of this split is to focus on movements rather than selected muscle groups.

Push is the action moving away from the body; trains the chest and shoulders.

Pull is the the action bringing towards the body; trains the back, abs and obliques.

Legs involve 'pushing' when training the quadriceps and 'pulling' when training the hamstrings. Legs are worked in one session due to the physical demands.

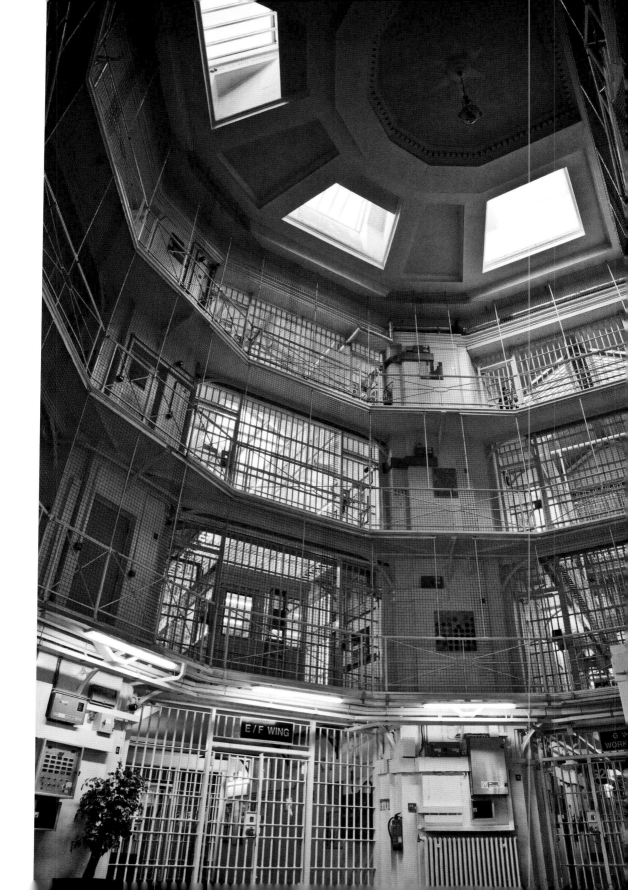

CARDIOVASCULAR TRAINING

LOW INTENSITY, LONG DURATION

This is aerobic training, working at an intensity of around 50-60% target heart rate (THR) of your maximum heart rate (MHR). Your rating of percieved exertion (RPE) should be around 6-10 of intensity. This is either marching or jogging slowly, easy and continuously over a long period of 40+ minutes. It is the least demanding form of aerobic exercise. In the workouts this is referred to as 'Rhythm' session.

Rhythm sessions aim not only to flush out the hard work of the day before but also to keep the body in the rhythm of exercise. Jogging at an easy/comfortable pace helps the body to get rid of any stiffness and soreness, whilst still improving endurance and aerobic capacity. It also better prepares the body for the next day of training.

MODERATE INTENSITY, MEDIUM DURATION

This is aerobic training, working at an intensity of around 60-80% THR. This is either jogging or running, at a moderate intensity over a medium period of 20-40 minutes. Your RPE should be around 10-14 of intensity. When running consistently, effort should be 60-70% THR. However, when running at intervals, effort should be 70-80% THR. In the workouts this is referred to as 'Tempo' session.

Tempo sessions are designed to be run at a challenging pace, which is manageable for a longer time. The session is used as a way of building up stamina and enables the body to work for longer, with more oxygen intake.

HIGH INTENSITY, SHORT DURATION

This is aerobic training, working at an intensity of around 80-90% THR. At 85% THR it is considered to be the anaerobic threshold. Your RPE should be around 15-19 of intensity. This is either running or sprinting at a high intensity over a short period of 5-20 minutes. In the workouts this is referred to as 'Lactic' session.

Lactic sessions are designed to improve your lactate threshold. This is where the body creates lactic acid because the muscles are not receiving enough oxygen for the exercise they are doing. This results in the body producing the chemical lactic acid which creates a burning feeling within the muscles being used. Lactic threshold exercise aims to delay the onset of lactic acid and therefore means that the body can exercise for longer without becoming tired.

ANAEROBIC INTERVAL TRAINING

This is anaerobic training, working at an intensity of around 90-100% THR. This is sprinting at maximum effort for a matter of seconds. Your RPE should be around 20, which is maximum exertion. In the workouts this is referred to as 'Speed' session.

Speed sessions are designed to make the body work as hard as possible for a short amount of time and burn excess fat. Includes a full recovery after each rep and improves the anaerobic fitness by improving power and increasing the fast twitch fibres in the body.

FARTLEK TRAINING

This involves both aerobic and anaerobic training at varied intensities. When working hard you will be about 70-100% THR and around 30-50% THR during recovery. Your RPE will vary from 6-18 of intensity. It is a flexible form of interval or continuous training, with no set time for intensity and speed during one session, over a period of 20-40 minutes. It will allow your body to recover between bursts of high intensity activity.

CARDIOVASCULAR TRAINING GUIDELINES

Variables	Low Intensity, Long Duration	Moderate Intensity, Medium Duration	High Intensity, Short Duration	Anaerobic Interval Training	Fartlek
Intensity	Low 50-60%	Moderate 60-80%	High 80-90%	Vigorous 90-100%	Low/ Vigorous 30-100%
Set duration (minutes)	N/A	N/A	N/A	1-2	N/A
Rest between sets (minutes)	N/A	N/A	N/A	1-5	N/A
Sets per exercise	1	1	1	5+	1
Duration (minutes)	40+	20-40	5-20	5-15	20-40
Frequency (per week)	5+	5+	3+	3+	4+
Method	March/Jog	Jog/Run	Run/Sprint	Sprint	Various

There is more information on cardiovascular training at the beginning of the Cardio chapter on page 41.

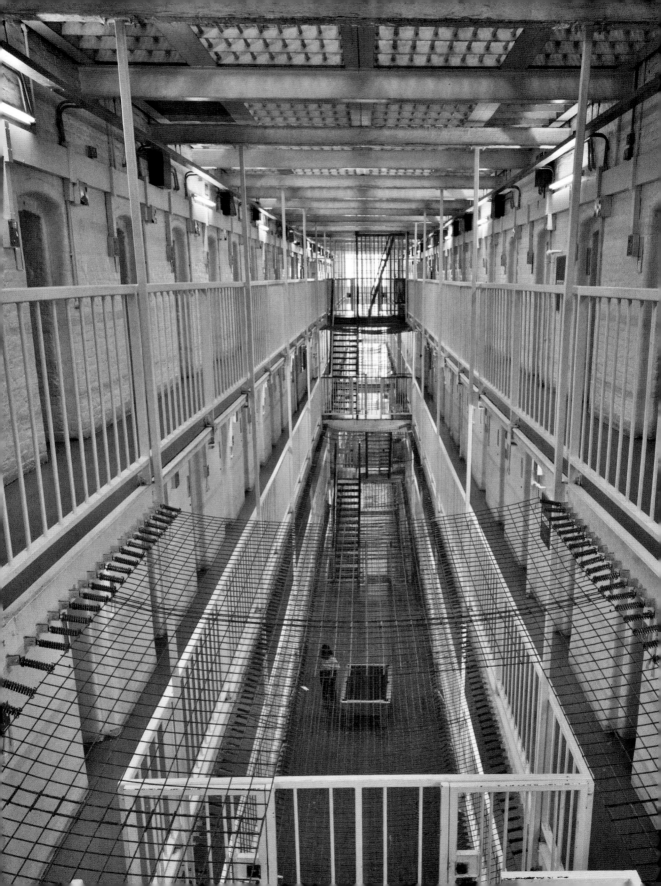

FLEXIBILITY TRAINING

Flexibility can be defined as the range of movement about a joint or series of joints and the length of muscles that cross the joints to assist freedom of movement.

Flexibility will vary between individuals mainly depending on the length of multi-joint muscles. Stretching is the main method to maintain or improve flexibility. You should stretch when your muscles are warm and body temperature is raised.

Increased flexibility will help avoid fatiguing the working muscles (agonist) and if the opposing muscles (antagonist) are more flexible, then the working muscle will not need to work as hard. Lack of muscle flexibility could result in muscle damage, joint stiffness and poor circulation.

There are two methods of stretching: Active (see Warm Up) and Passive (see Cool Down). Although stretching should always be included in a workout, it has benefits in its own right.

FLEXIBILITY TRAINING GUIDELINES

Variables	Active Stretching	Passive Stretching
Intensity	Low	Low
Reps	12+	15-30 secs
Rest between sets	N/A	N/A
Sets per exercise	1-2	1-4
Duration	10-15 mins	10-15 mins
Frequency	5+ per week	5+ per week
Method	Mobilisation	Static maintenance and development stretches

ACTIVE STRETCHING

This method of stretching activates and warms up the muscles without using any other assistance. Mobilisation, also known as dynamic stretching, is a form of active stretching and is an important part of a warm up.

There is more information and the benefits of active stretching at the beginning of the Mobilisation chapter page 27.

WARM UP

The aim is to prepare the cardiovascular, respiratory and neuromuscular system for the exercise to follow.

The warm up will:

Raise your heart rate.
Raise your breathing rate.
Raise your muscle temperature.
Stretch muscles and mobilise joints appropriate for the exercise to follow.

Step 1: Start by either flexing and extending; abducting and adducting; rotating clockwise and anti-clockwise at the following joints for 10 reps each.

Fingers
Wrists
Elbows
Shoulders
Neck
Trunk and shoulder blades
Hips
Knees
Ankles
Feet and toes

Step 2: Once you have warmed up your joints you should then move on to either marching or jogging on the spot. This is a good way to gently raise your heart and breathing rate and muscle temperature. Continue for 5 minutes.

Step 3: You are now ready to mobilise your muscles and limbs. Perform 1-2 mobilisation stretches per main muscle group that you are about to work. If a particular muscle group feels stiff or sore then perform a static stretch for that muscle group.

A warm up should last about 10-15 minutes.

PASSIVE STRETCHING

This method of stretching is achieved with assistance from an external source (held by yourself, wall or partner) in order to increase the muscle length and joint range. This is done using static stretches and there are two types: static maintenance and static development and is usually associated with a cool down.

There is more information and the benefits of passive stretching at the beginning of the Static Stretching chapter page 177.

COOL DOWN

The aim is to bring the body and mind back to the level before exercise was undertaken.

The cool down will:

Decrease your heart rate.
Decrease your breathing.
Decrease your muscles temperature.
Stretch muscles in an appropriate manner.

Step 1: Jogging is a good way to reduce your heart rate at a steady pace. After intense exercise, blood is diverted to the working muscles. Light movements using muscles that have been used during the session will help remove lactic acid and prevent blood pooling. Continue for 5 minutes. Follow this with passive stretching.

Step 2: You are now ready to perform static stretches to stretch out the muscles and limbs used during your workout.

Static maintenance stretches – stretch the muscles until you feel tension, but not so as you feel pain, maintain good posture and alignment throughout the stretch. Hold until you feel the muscle tension reduce, usually 15-20 seconds. Relax and repeat the stretch if needed.

Static development stretches – repeat the above process, performing each stretch 3-4 times more, increasing the range of movement each time until you feel tension. Hold until tension reduces.

A cool down should last just as long as a warm up, about 10-15 minutes.

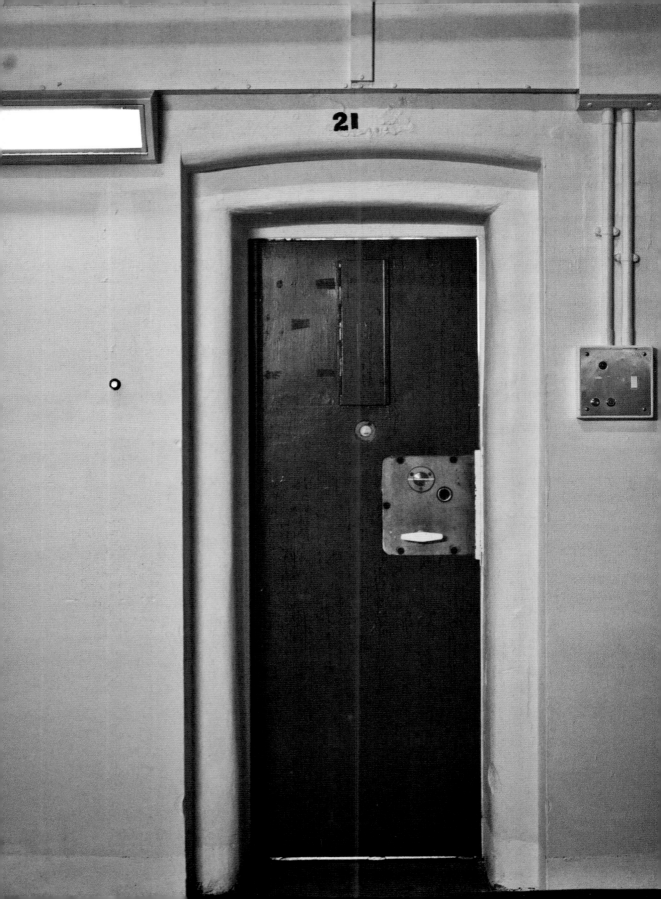

MOBILISATION

Mobilisation or dynamic stretching exercises are forms of active stretching. They are stretches performed while moving, without any other assistance. This form of stretching will mobilise, stretch and increase the range of movement of the muscles and limbs.

The purpose is to stimulate the muscles, tendons, nervous system and joints. Mobilisation will help bring your body from a state of rest and prepare it for physical activity as part of a warm up.

Performing appropriate mobilisation stretches can have a big impact on your workout, as it will allow your body to move more efficiently. The stretches should be specific to the workout to follow, with similar actions and working the same muscles that will be used.

Begin slowly and as your mobility improves, gradually increase the speed and range of movement to make the exercises more dynamic. Remember to stay within your own normal range of movement, but work to gradually increase the range and speed as you progress.

Stretching will lengthen the muscles, reduce muscle tension and increase the normal range of movement. This will in turn increase the distance the limbs can move before they are put under strain. Increased distance will result in more power and therefore improve ability and performance.

Mobilisation is an important part of the warm up, for injury prevention and performance improvement. If not performed you are at a higher risk of injury.

NECK FLEXION AND EXTENSION

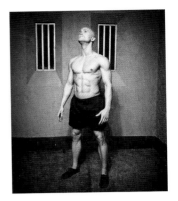

Target Muscle Groups
Primary: Trapezius, Rhomboids
Secondary:

Step 1: Stand with your shoulders relaxed, feet shoulder-width apart, arms by your sides and your spine in a neutral position.

Step 2: Extend your neck forwards and slowly raise your chin to look up to the ceiling.

Step 3: Continue the movement, lowering your head down and tuck your chin in towards your chest.

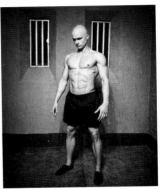

Tip: This exercise is good for preventing neck stiffness. It can also be performed seated.

NECK ROTATION

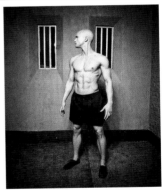

Target Muscle Groups
Primary: Trapezius
Secondary:

Step 1: Stand with your shoulders relaxed, feet shoulder-width apart, arms by your sides and your spine in a neutral position.

Step 2: Turn your head round slowly to one side to look over your shoulder.

Step 3: Continue the movement, looking over the opposite shoulder.

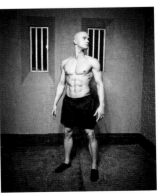

Tip: Good for neck aches and promotes flexibility.

LATERAL NECK FLEXION

Target Muscle Groups
Primary: Deltoids
Secondary: Rhomboids, Trapezius

Step 1: Stand with your shoulders relaxed, feet shoulder-width apart, arms by your sides and your spine in a neutral position.

Step 2: Facing ahead, tilt your head to one side, lowering your ear down towards your shoulder, keeping your chin up.

Step 3: Continue the movement, tilting your head to the other side.

Tip: Good for aching muscles in the neck and upper back, bad sleeping position and posture.

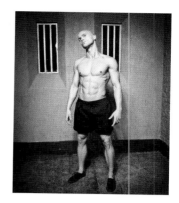

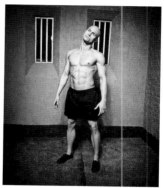

SIDE TO FRONT CROSSOVER

Target Muscle Groups
Primary: Deltoids, Pectorals
Secondary: Rhomboids, Trapezius

Step 1: Stand with your shoulders relaxed, feet shoulder-width apart, arms extended out to the sides at shoulder-height and your spine in a neutral position.

Step 2: Looking forwards, bring your arms straight in to cross over in front of your chest.

Step 3: Continue the movement, uncrossing your arms, taking them back out to the sides, keeping them at shoulder-height throughout the movement. Swap the upper and lower positions of the arms as they cross over.

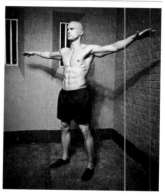

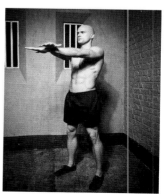

ARM CIRCLE

Target Muscle Groups
Primary: Deltoids
Secondary: Trapezius, Pectorals,
Latissimus Dorsi

Step 1: Stand with your shoulders relaxed, feet shoulder-width apart, arms by your sides and your spine in a neutral position.

Step 2: Keeping your arms straight, rotate them in a circular motion. Widen the circles as your shoulders become more mobile.

Step 3: Continue the movement, rotating your arms in the opposite direction.

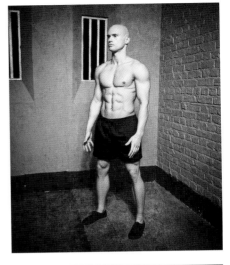

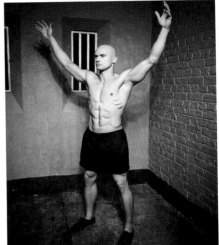

Tips: This exercise warms up the muscles in the shoulders, gets your joints moving and blood circulating.

For variation, rotate one arm forwards and one backwards.

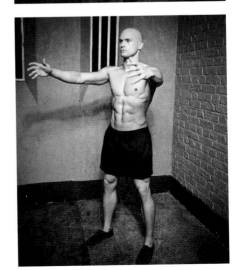

TORSO PUSH AND PULL

Target Muscle Groups

Primary: Pectorals, Trapezius, Rhomboids

Secondary: Deltoids, Latissimus Dorsi

Step 1: Stand with your shoulders relaxed and feet shoulder-width apart. Extend your arms straight out in front at shoulder-height with palms facing forwards. Round your upper back, dropping your chest slightly forwards.

Step 2: Bend your elbows as you pull your arms back. Raise and open your chest, squeezing your shoulder blades. Arch your lower back slightly.

Step 3: Continue the movement, pushing your arms forwards and pulling them back.

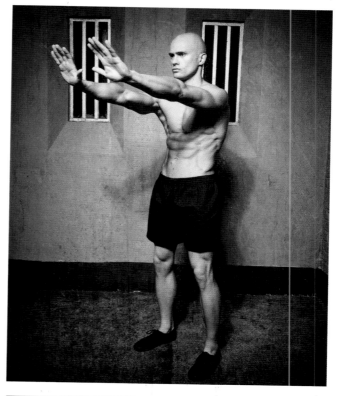

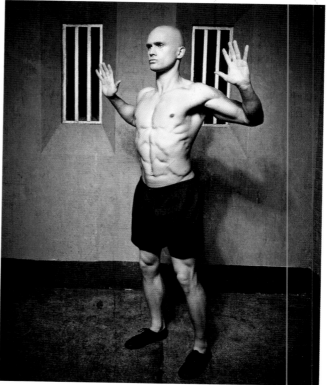

TORSO ROTATION

Target Muscle Groups
Primary: Abdominals, Obliques, Erector Spinae
Secondary:

Step 1: Stand with your shoulders relaxed and feet shoulder-width apart. With elbows bent out to the sides, hold your hands up in front of your chest, palms down and fingers touching.

Step 2: Keeping your hips facing forwards, twist at the waist to rotate your upper body round to one side.

Step 3: Continue the movement, rotating to the other side, with your hips facing forwards throughout.

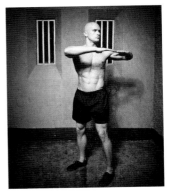

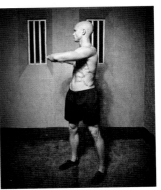

LATERAL TORSO FLEXION

Target Muscle Groups
Primary: Obliques, Abdominals
Secondary: Latissimus Dorsi

Step 1: Stand with your shoulders relaxed, feet shoulder-width apart, arms by your sides and your spine in a neutral position.

Step 2: Engage your abdominals and bend at the waist to one side, sliding your hand down your leg.

Step 3: Continue the movement, bending down to the other side.

Tip: As you bend to the side, avoid leaning forwards or backwards.

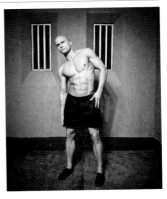

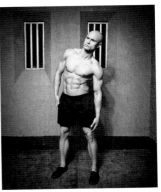

ROLL UP

Target Muscle Groups
Primary: Erector Spine, Gluteals, Hamstrings
Secondary: Rhomboids

Step 1: With your feet shoulder-width apart, bend forward at the hips, hanging your arms and upper body down towards the floor.

Step 2: Keep your shoulders and neck relaxed as you slowly roll up, uncurling your spine until you are in an upright standing position.

Step 3: Continue the movement, slowly curl your spine back down towards the floor.

Tip: Keep your abdominals engaged throughout the movement to protect your lower back.

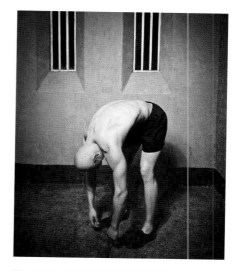

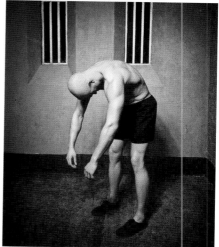

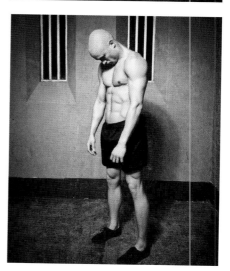

HIP CIRCLE

Target Muscle Groups
Primary: Abdominals, Obliques, Erector Spinae
Secondary: Gluteals

Step 1: Stand with your shoulders relaxed, feet shoulder-width apart, hands on your hips and your spine in a neutral position.

Step 2: Looking forwards, circle your hips in a continuous motion. Widen the circles as your hips become more mobile.

Step 3: Continue the movement, circling in the opposite direction.

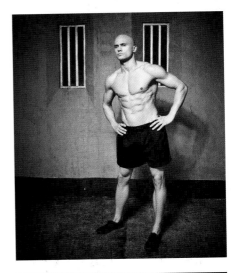

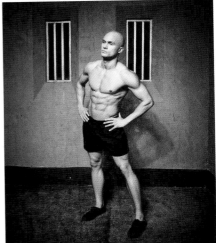

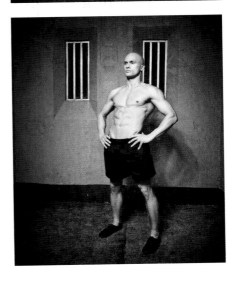

HIP TWIST

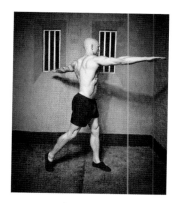

Target Muscle Groups
Primary: Deltoids, Abdominals, Obliques, Erector Spinae
Secondary: Gluteals

Step 1: Stand with your arms extended out to the sides at shoulder-height and your feet wider than shoulder-width apart.

Step 2: Twist at the waist to rotate your upper body and hips to one side. Shift your weight onto that foot as you raise the heel of your back foot.

Step 3: Continue the movement, twisting to the other side.

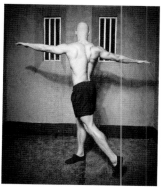

HIP SWIVEL

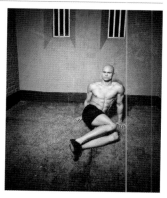

Target Muscle Groups
Primary: Quadriceps, Obliques
Secondary: Gluteals

Step 1: Sit with your hands behind you for support. Bend your knees and place your feet together, flat on the floor, in front of you.

Step 2: Keeping your upper body still, lower both knees down to one side.

Step 3: Continue the movement, raising your knees back up to the centre and lowering to the other side.

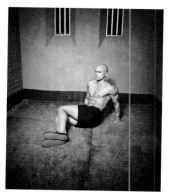

FRONT LEG SWING

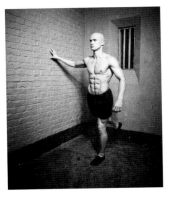

Target Muscle Groups
Primary: Quadriceps, Gluteals
Secondary: Hamstrings, Abdominals

Step 1: Stand with a wall to one side, holding on for balance. Keep a slight bend in your supporting leg.

Step 2: Swing the other leg backwards, keeping your upper body straight.

Step 3: Continue the movement, swinging your leg forwards. Repeat, then alternate with the opposite leg.

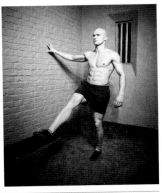

Tip: This exercise mobilises the hip joint.

SIDE LEG SWING

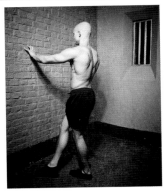

Target Muscle Groups
Primary: Adductors, Gluteals
Secondary: Quadriceps, Hamstrings, Abdominals

Step 1: Stand facing a wall, with your feet hip-width apart. Place your palms flat against the wall at shoulder-height.

Step 2: Swing your leg out to the side, keeping your upper body straight.

Step 3: Continue the movement, swinging your leg across your body. Repeat, then alternate with the opposite leg.

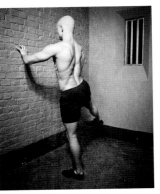

Tip: This exercise mobilises the muscles in the gluteals and groin area.

LEG STEP OVER

Target Muscle Groups

Primary: Quadriceps, Gluteals, Adductors

Secondary: Hamstrings, Abdominals

Step 1: Stand with a wall to one side, holding on for balance. Raise your leg out to the side, with a slight bend.

Step 2: Raise the leg up and inwards, in a stepping action and lower down towards the floor.

Step 3: Continue the movement, raising your leg back up and outwards. Repeat, then alternate with the opposite leg.

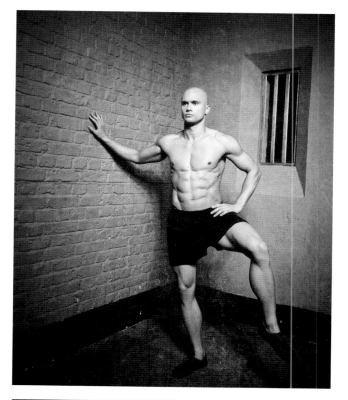

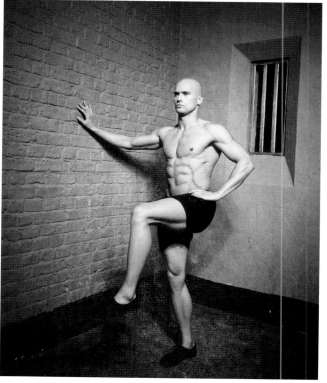

HIGH LUNGE

Target Muscle Groups
Primary: Quadriceps, Hamstrings, Adductors
Secondary: Gluteals

Step 1: In a downward facing position, place your hands slightly wider than shoulder-width apart. Extend your legs straight behind you, with your feet hip-width apart, toes tucked under and heels pushed away.

Step 2: Maintaining a straight back, step one foot forwards and place next to the outside of your hand. Lean forwards with your hips to feel the stretch in your inner thighs.

Step 3: Continue the movement, stepping your foot back. Repeat with the opposite leg.

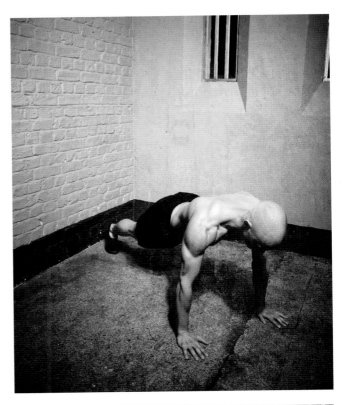

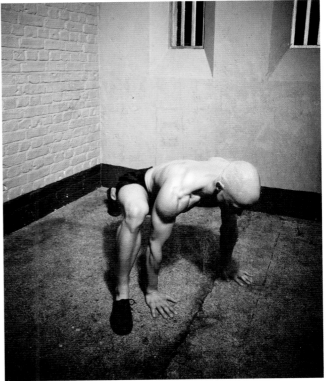

DOUBLE CALF RAISE

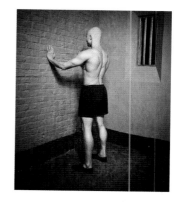

Target Muscle Groups
Primary: Gastrocnemius, Sloeus
Secondary:

Step 1: Stand facing a wall with feet hip-width apart. Place your palms flat against the wall at shoulder-height.

Step 2: Raise your heels, placing your weight on the balls of your feet.

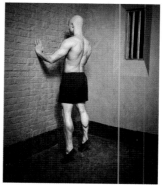

Step 3: Continue the movement, lowering your heels back down and without touching the floor raise back up. Increase the tempo as you perform the exercise.

Tip: This exercise can be performed single leg.

CALF PRESS OUT

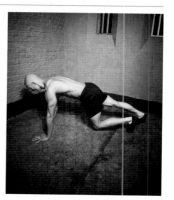

Target Muscle Groups
Primary: Gastrocnemius, Soleus
Secondary:

Step 1: In a downward facing position, place your hands slightly wider than shoulder-width apart. Extend your legs straight behind you with your feet hip-width apart, toes tucked under and heels pushed away.

Step 2: Raise your hips slightly, bend one knee and straighten the other leg, as you push the heel of the straight leg towards the floor.

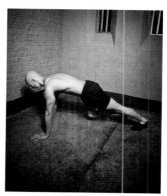

Step 3: Continue the movement, alternating sides.

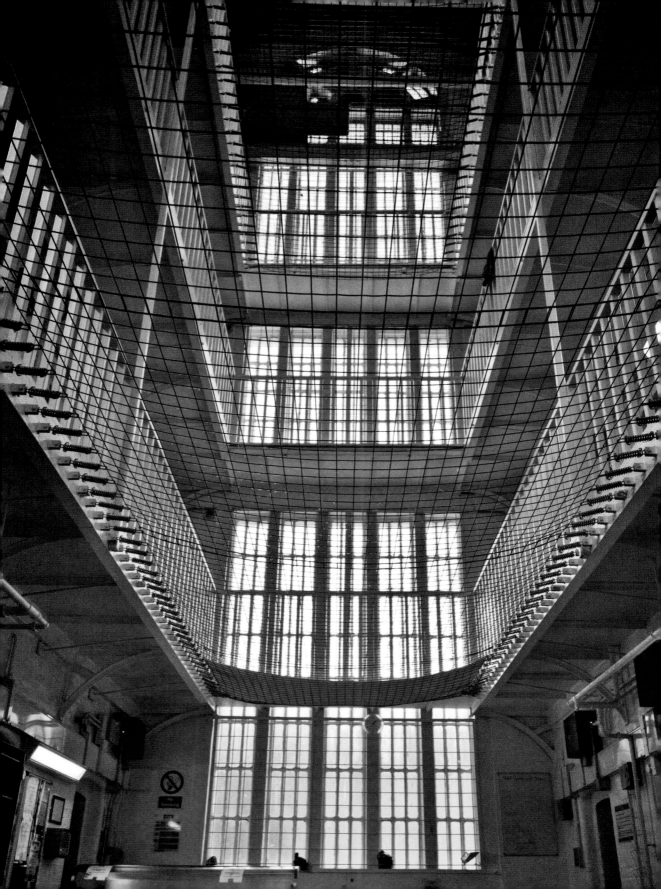

CARDIO

Cardiovascular exercise, also known as aerobic exercise, is any exercise that increases the heart and respiration rates while using large muscle groups repetitively and rhythmically. The heart is a muscle, whose function is to pump blood around the body. Working the heart will make it stronger and more efficient.

The energy needed for cardio exercise is provided by the oxygenated blood that is being pumped around the body, the cardiovascular system. Walking, running, sprinting, biking, rowing and swimming are all forms of cardiovascular exercise. Cardio activity can be low to high intensity.

Endurance exercise, carried out for a long duration, such as walking and running, is called aerobic exercise. Exercise that is carried out for a short duration, requiring a short powerful burst of high intensity exertion, such as sprinting, is called anaerobic exercise.

Plyometric exercises combine cardiovascular and toning exercises. They increase muscular endurance and power. Plyometric exercises, such as jumping and bounding involve rapid, repeated muscle changes from stretched to contracted positions.

Regular cardio exercise, 20 minutes or more on most days will improve heart function, strengthen muscles, improve circulation, reduce blood pressure and increase energy and stamina levels.

Increasing the amount of cardio exercise will improve cardiovascular endurance, burn calories, loose fat and build muscle mass.

Regular cardiovascular exercise will lower the risk of many diseases such as heart disease, high blood pressure and high cholesterol. Weight bearing cardio exercise is good for maintaining healthy bones, as well as conditioning the heart.

Cardiovascular exercise is known to improve health generally, reduce stress and have a positive effect on mental health.

JOG ON THE SPOT

Target Muscle Groups

Primary: Quadriceps, Gluteals, Hamstrings

Secondary: Gastrocnemius, Soleus, Deltoids

Step 1: Stand with your feet hip-width apart and arms by your sides. Keep your back straight and head up.

Step 2: Begin to lightly jog on the spot, lifting your knees high. Alternate your arms in a controlled swing, with bent elbows, as you jog.

Step 3: Continue this movement.

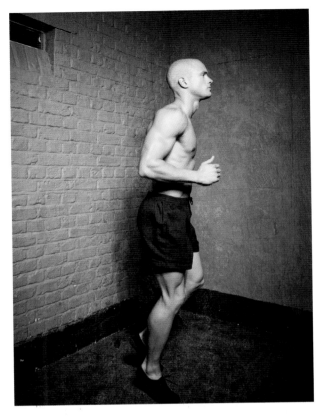

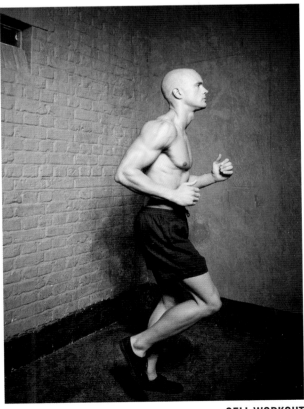

CELL WORKOUT

SPRINT ON THE SPOT

Target Muscle Groups

Primary: Quadriceps, Gluteals, Hamstrings

Secondary: Gastrocnemius, Soleus, Deltoids, Biceps

Step 1: Stand with your feet hip-width apart and arms by your sides. Keep your back straight and head up.

Step 2: Begin by running on the spot, then gradually increase your speed until you are sprinting. Pump your arms as fast as you can and lift your knees up to your chest, high and fast. Keep your abdominals engaged.

Step 3: Continue this movement.

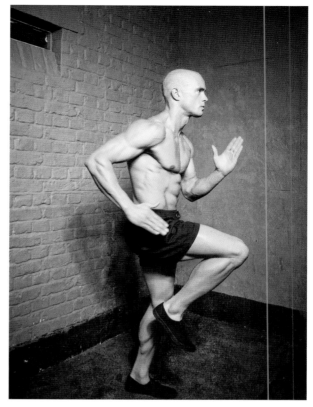

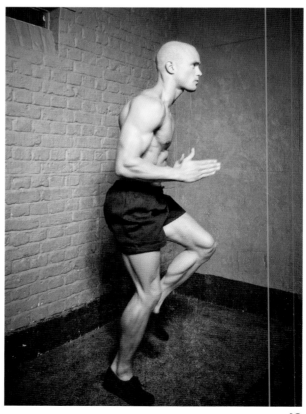

GLUTE KICKER

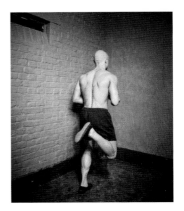

Target Muscle Groups
Primary: Quadriceps, Gluteus, Hamstrings
Secondary: Gastrocnemius, Soleus

Step 1: Stand with your feet hip-width apart. Keep your back straight and head up.

Step 2: Begin by jogging on the spot, bringing your heels up high behind you to touch your glutes. Keep your arms slightly bent to aid balance.

Step 3: Continue this movement, increasing the speed.

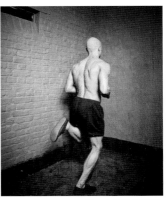

HIGH KNEES

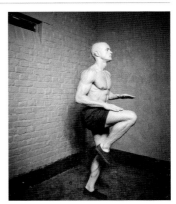

Target Muscle Groups
Primary: Quadriceps, Gluteals, Hamstrings
Secondary: Gastrocnemius, Soleus

Step 1: Stand with your feet shoulder-width apart and arms slightly bent in front of you, with palms facing down. Keep your back straight and head up.

Step 2: Jog on the spot, lifting your knees up high in front of you, touching your hands as they come up.

Step 3: Continue this movement, increasing the speed and height of your knees.

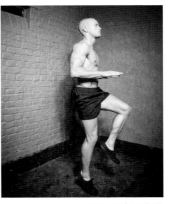

POWER KNEE STRIKE

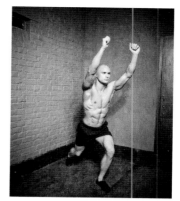

Target Muscle Groups
Primary: Quadriceps, Gluteals, Hamstrings
Secondary: Deltoids, Abdominals

Step 1: Stand with feet hip-width apart and your arms extended straight overhead.

Step 2: Engage your abdominals. Place your weight on one leg and bend the knee of the other leg and bring it up towards your chest. At the same time pull your arms down straight by your sides.

Step 3: Continue the movement, extending your arms and leg back to the start position, tapping your toe lightly on the floor. Repeat with the opposite leg.

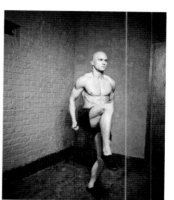

POWER KNEE STRIKE WITH TWIST

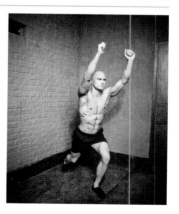

Target Muscle Groups
Primary: Quadriceps, Gluteals, Hamstring
Secondary: Deltoids, Obliques, Abdominals

Step 1: Stand with feet hip-width apart and your arms extended straight overhead.

Step 2: Engage your abdominals. Place your weight on one leg and bend the knee of the other leg and bring it up and across your chest. At the same time twist at the waist as you pull your arms across and down to the outside of the thigh of the leg that is lifted.

Step 3: Continue the movement, extending your arms and leg back to the start position, tapping your toe lightly on the floor. Repeat with the opposite leg.

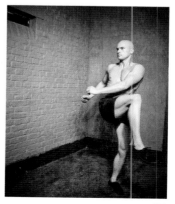

SQUAT THRUST

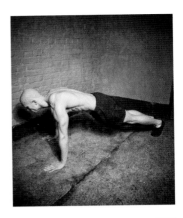

Target Muscle Groups
Primary: Quadriceps, Gluteus, Hamstrings
Secondary: Deltoids, Triceps, Abdominals

Step 1: In a downward facing position, place your hands slightly wider than shoulder-width apart. Extend your legs straight behind you, with your feet hip-width apart, toes tucked under and heels pushed away.

Step 2: Looking down, press down through your hands and shift your weight onto them as you bend your knees to thrust your legs in under your chest. Keep your abdominals engaged.

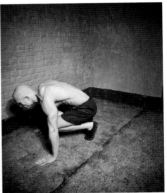

Step 3: Continue the movement, explosively thrusting your legs back to the start position, with your arms straight.

ALTERNATING SQUAT THRUST

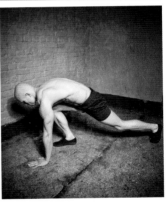

Target Muscle Groups
Primary: Quadriceps, Gluteals, Hamstrings
Secondary: Deltoids, Triceps, Abdominals

Step 1: In a downward facing position, place your hands slightly wider than shoulder-width apart. Extend your legs straight behind you, with your feet hip-width apart, toes tucked under and heels pushed away.

Step 2: Looking down, bend one knee to thrust the leg inwards towards your chest. Keep your abdominals engaged.

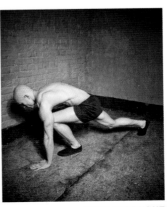

Step 3: Continue the movement, explosively alternating the legs, thrusting the bent leg back out and at the same time bringing the other leg in under your chest.

SQUAT THRUST WITH SINGLE LEG

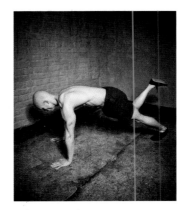

Target Muscle Groups
Primary: Quadriceps, Gluteals, Hamstrings
Secondary: Deltoids, Triceps, Abdominals

Step 1: In a downward facing position, place your hands slightly wider than shoulder-width apart. Extend your legs straight behind you, with your feet hip-width apart and lift one foot off the floor.

Step 2: Looking down, bend the knee as you thrust the supporting leg inwards towards your chest, transferring your weight onto your hands. Keep the raised leg off the floor. Keep your abdominals engaged.

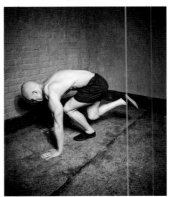

Step 3: Continue the movement, explosively thrusting the leg back out. Repeat with the opposite leg.

SUMO SQUAT THRUST

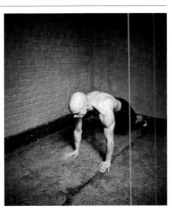

Target Muscle Groups
Primary: Quadriceps, Gluteals, Hamstrings, Adductors **Secondary:** Deltoids, Triceps, Abdominals
Step 1: In a downward facing position, place your hands slightly wider than shoulder-width apart. Extend your legs straight behind you, with your feet slightly wider than hip-width apart, toes tucked under and heels pushed away.

Step 2: Looking down, press down through your hands and shift your weight onto them as you bend your knees to thrust your legs forward, taking your feet to the outside of your hands.

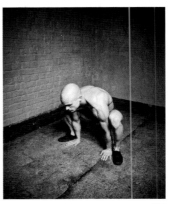

Step 3: Continue the movement, explosively thrusting your legs back to the start position, with your arms straight.

JUMPING JACK

Target Muscle Groups

Primary: Quadriceps, Gluteals, Hamstrings, Adductors

Secondary: Gastrocnemius, Soleus, Deltoids

Step 1: Stand with your feet shoulder-width apart and your hands by your sides.

Step 2: Jump up a few inches in the air, and land with your feet wider than shoulder-width apart. At the same time extend your arms straight out and up to 45-degrees above shoulder-height so that you are forming a star shape.

Step 3: Continue the movement, jumping up again to return back to the start position, bringing your arms and legs back in. Stay light on your toes.

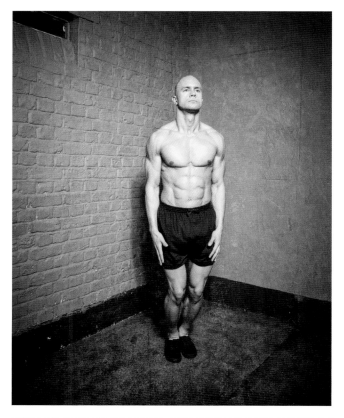

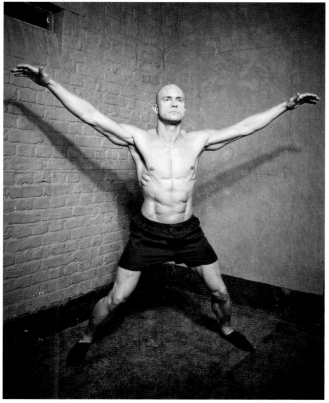

JUMPING CROSS JACK

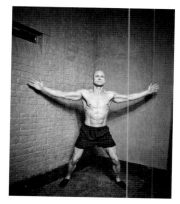

Target Muscle Groups
Primary: Quadriceps, Gluteals, Hamstrings, Adductors
Secondary: Gastrocnemius, Soleus, Deltoids

Step 1: Stand with your feet out wide and your arms extended out straight to 45-degrees above shoulder-height to form a star shape.

Step 2: Jump in, crossing one foot in front of the other. Bring your arms in straight overhead, crossing one hand in front of the other.

Step 3: Continue the movement, jumping back out to the star shape keeping light on your toes. Repeat, alternating which arm and foot crosses in front.

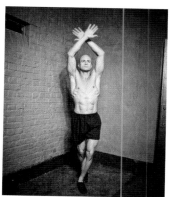

JUMPING FRONT CROSS JACK

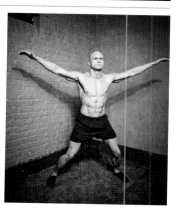

Target Muscle Groups
Primary: Quadriceps, Gluteals, Hamstrings, Adductors
Secondary: Gastrocnemius, Soleus, Deltoids

Step 1: Stand with your feet more than hip-width apart and your arms straight out to the sides at shoulder-height.

Step 2: Jump up and cross your arms in front of your chest while crossing one leg in front of the other.

Step 3: Continue the movement, jumping back out. Repeat, alternating your arm and foot positions as you jump back in.

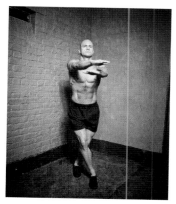

PENDULUM LEG SWING

Target Muscle Groups
Primary: Quadriceps, Gluteals, Hamstrings, Adductors
Secondary: Abdominals

Step 1: Stand with your feet together and hands on your hips.

Step 2: Maintain a straight back and engage your abdominals. Swing one leg straight out to the side to a 45-degree angle.

Step 3: Continue the movement, bringing the leg back down to the centre and at the same time, swing the opposite leg out to the side.

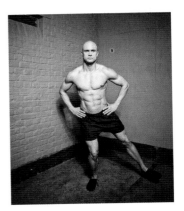

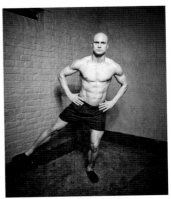

LATERAL TOE TAP

Target Muscle Groups
Primary: Quadriceps, Gluteals, Hamstrings, Adductors
Secondary: Abdominals

Step 1: Stand with your feet slightly apart and hands on your hips. Bend your knees and tilt forward slightly at the hips.

Step 2: Maintaining a straight back, toe tap one foot lightly out to the side.

Step 3: Continue the movement, quickly return that foot to the centre position. Repeat, tapping the other foot out to the side.

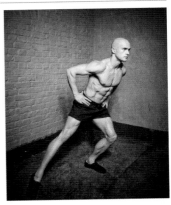

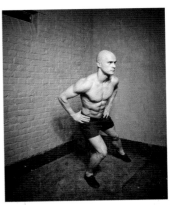

CELL WORKOUT

PLYO IN OUT SQUAT JUMP

Target Muscle Groups

Primary: Quadriceps, Gluteals, Hamstrings, Adductors

Secondary: Gastrocnemius, Soleus

Step 1: Stand with your feet close together and hands up in front of your chest, elbows bent. Tilt forwards slightly at the hips.

Step 2: Maintain a straight back as you jump both feet out into a wide lowered squat position.

Step 3: Continue the movement, jumping both feet back together and landing into a narrow squat.

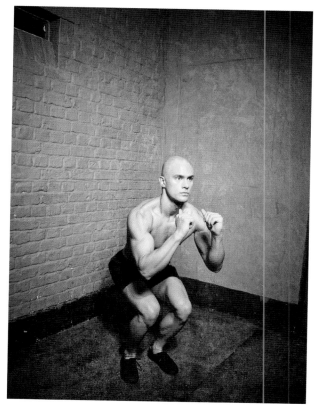

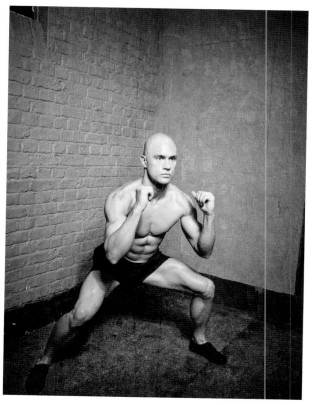

PLYO POWER SKIP

Target Muscle Groups

Primary: Quadriceps, Gluteals, Hamstrings

Secondary: Gastrocnemius, Soleus, Abdominals

Step 1: Stand with feet shoulder-width apart and arms slightly bent. Keep your back straight and head up, looking straight ahead.

Step 2: Raise one knee up towards your chest in an explosive skipping action, with both feet leaving the floor. Keeping arms bent, raise the opposite arm upwards and forwards and the other arm upwards and backwards.

Step 3: Continue the movement, alternating your knee and arm positions and gradually increasing your speed, to reach a high skipping movement, landing on the balls of your feet each time they touch the ground.

Tip: This can also be performed moving forwards and backwards.

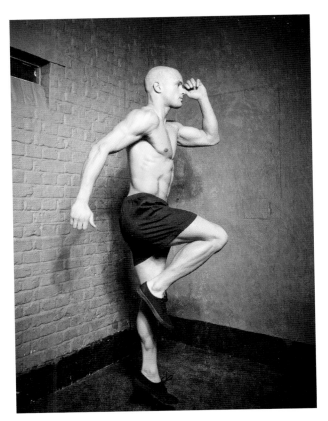

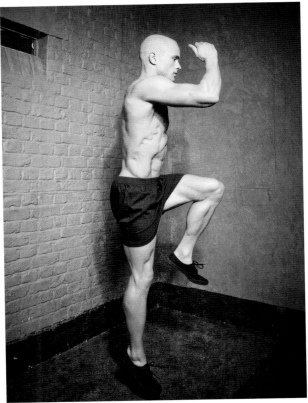

SPOTTY DOG

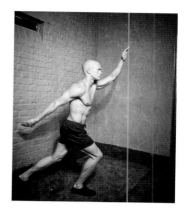

Target Muscle Groups
Primary: Quadriceps, Gluteals, Hamstrings
Secondary: Gastrocnemius, Soleus, Deltoids

Step 1: Stand with one leg in front of the other, in a staggered stance. Maintain straight arms and hold the opposite arm to the front leg at a 45-degree angle. Hold your other arm straight back.

Step 2: Explosively jump off the floor and alternate the leg positions, at the same time switching arm positions.

Step 3: Continue the movement, alternating your arm and leg positions each time you are in the air.

Tip: Keep your stride distance short, so that your knee does not go too far forward.

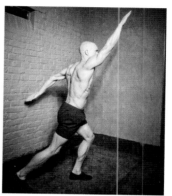

ANKLE HOP

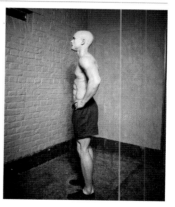

Target Muscle Groups
Primary: Gastronemius, Solues
Secondary:

Step 1: Stand with your hands on your hips. Keep your back straight and head up.

Step 2: Explosively hop up using the force from your ankles and calves, with little bend in the knee.

Step 3: Continue the movement.

Tips: When performing this exercise, imagine you are jumping over a skipping rope. Can also be performed single leg.

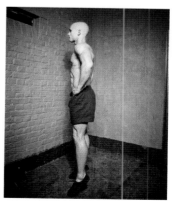

PLYO SQUAT JUMP

Target Muscle Groups
Primary: Quadriceps, Gluteals, Hamstrings
Secondary: Gastrocnemius, Soleus

Step 1: Stand with feet slightly wider than shoulder-width apart and arms extended out straight in front of your chest.

Step 2: Bend at the knees to lower yourself into a squat, until your thighs are parallel to the floor, then explosively jump up.

Step 3: Continue the movement, decelerating with soft knees as you lower into a squat.

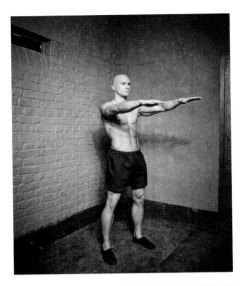

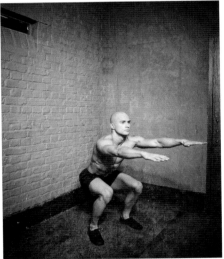

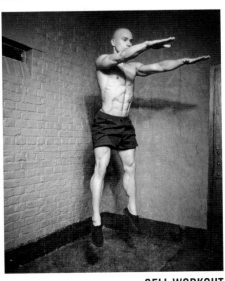

PLYO VERTICAL ROCKET JUMP

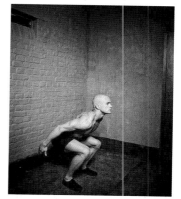

Target Muscle Groups
Primary: Quadriceps, Gluteals, Hamstrings, Deltoids
Secondary: Gastrocnemius, Soleus

Step 1: Stand with feet slightly wider than shoulder-width apart and arms down by your sides.

Step 2: Bend at the knees to lower yourself into a squat, until your thighs are parallel to the floor, then explosively jump up, swinging your arms straight up above your head to power upwards.

Step 3: Continue the movement, decelerating with soft knees as you lower into a squat.

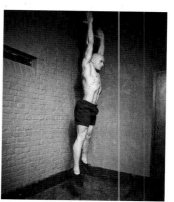

TUCK JUMP

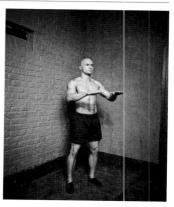

Target Muscle Groups
Primary: Quadriceps, Gluteals, Hamstrings
Secondary: Gastrocnemius, Soleus, Abdominals

Step 1: Stand with your knees slightly bent and feet shoulder-width apart. Bend your elbows so that your hands are up level with your chest, palms facing down and fingers pointed forwards.

Step 2: Explosively jump up, bringing your knees up towards your chest to touch your hands, to a tuck position.

Step 3: Continue the movement, landing on the balls of your feet with your knees soft and slightly bent, before jumping up again straightaway.

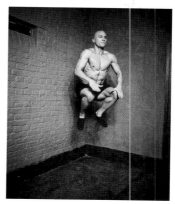

PLYO STAR JUMP

Target Muscle Groups

Primary: Quadriceps, Gluteals, Hamstrings, Adductors

Secondary: Gastrocnemius, Soleus, Deltoids

Step 1: Bend at the knees to lower yourself into a narrow squat, until your thighs are parallel to the floor and hands by your feet.

Step 2: Explosively jump up, raising your arms and legs outwards diagonally to form a star shape.

Step 3: Continue the movement, decelerating with soft knees as you lower into a squat while returning your hands to your feet.

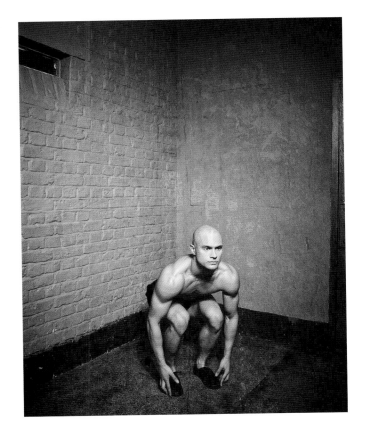

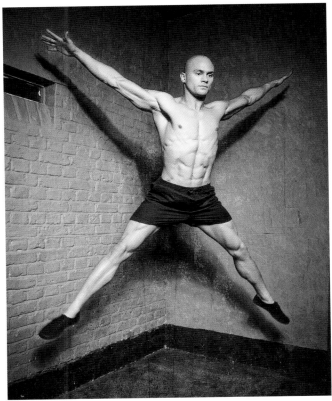

PLYO SERGEANT JUMP

Target Muscle Groups
Primary: Quadriceps, Gluteals, Hamstrings, Deltoids
Secondary: Gastrocnemius, Soleus

Step 1: Stand side on to a wall. Lower down in a squat position

Step 2: Jump straight up in the air, taking both feet off the floor, stretching one hand to touch the wall as high up as you can.

Step 3: Continue the movement, decelerating with soft knees as you bend into a squat. Repeat, then alternate with the opposite arm.

Tip: This is a difficult exercise. It is very good for developing explosive power in the lower body muscles.

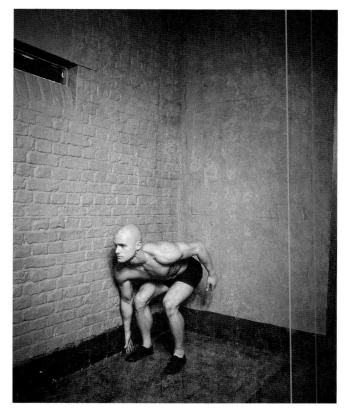

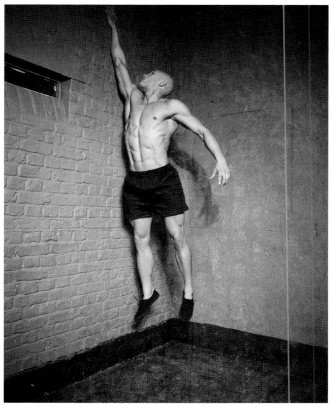

PLYO LATERAL SQUAT JUMP

Target Muscle Groups
Primary: Quadriceps, Gluteals, Hamstrings
Secondary: Gastrocnemius, Soleus

Step 1: From a standing position, bend at the knees to lower yourself into a squat, until your thighs are parallel to the floor. Bend your elbows to bring your hands up in front of your chest.

Step 2: Explosively jump up and to one side, using your arms to power upwards.

Step 3: Continue the movement, decelerating with soft knees as you bend into a squat. Repeat, jumping back to the start position.

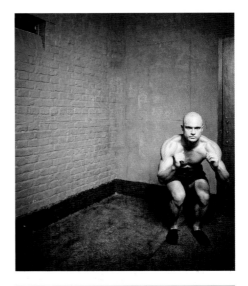

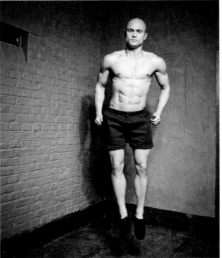

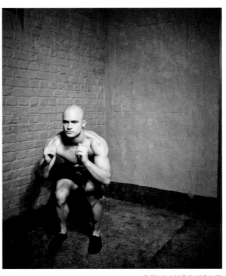

PLYO LATERAL BOUND

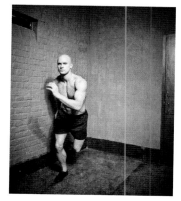

Target Muscle Groups
Primary: Quadriceps, Gluteals, Hamstrings, Adductors
Secondary: Gastrocnemius, Soleus

Step 1: From a standing position, raise one leg off the floor and bend at the knee to lower yourself into a half-squat. Bend your elbows and bring your hands up in front of your chest.

Step 2: Explosively hop out to the side, at the same time bending the other leg up behind. Alternate the arm swings.

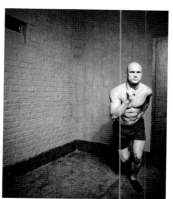

Step 3: Continue the movement, immediately hopping onto the other side, shifting your weight onto the opposite leg.

PLYO LATERAL TOUCH DOWN

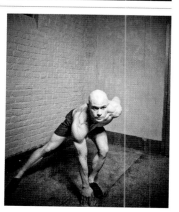

Target Muscle Groups
Primary: Quadriceps, Gluteals, Hamstrings, Adductors
Secondary: Gastrocnemius, Soleus

Step 1: Bend one knee and extend the other leg straight out to the side. Rotate your upper body and reach across and down to touch towards the foot of the bent leg with the opposite hand.

Step 2: Quickly jump up, swapping the positions of the legs, taking the bent leg straight out to the other side and bringing the extended leg into the centre, with knee bent. Reach across and touch down towards the foot of the bent leg with the opposite hand.

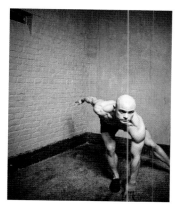

Step 3: Continue the movement, alternating the legs and rotating touch-downs to the centre.

PLYO BROAD JUMP

Target Muscle Groups
Primary: Quadriceps, Gluteals, Hamstrings, Deltoids
Secondary: Gastrocnemius, Soleus

Step 1: Stand with feet shoulder-width apart and arms raised overhead.

Step 2: Hinge forwards at the hips and bend your knees to lower your upper body down into a deep squat. Swing your arms back behind you. Swing your arms forwards, pushing down through your feet to extend the knees and hips to jump explosively up and forwards.

Step 3: Continue the movement, landing on both feet, decelerating as you bend your knees to lower into a squat, before returning to the upright standing position.

Tips: The broad jump is an effective exercise for developing explosive power. As a variation, you can reverse the movement.

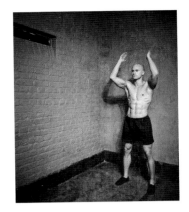
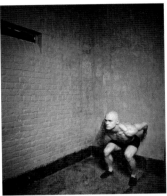
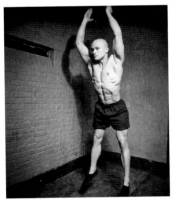
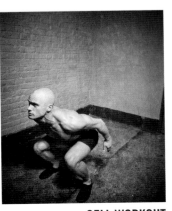

PLYO DIAGONAL BOUND

Target Muscle Groups

Primary: Quadriceps, Gluteals, Hamstrings, Adductors

Secondary: Gastrocnemius, Soleus, Deltoids

Step 1: From a standing position, raise one leg off the floor and bend at the knee to lower yourself into a half-squat. Bend your elbows and bring your hands up in front of your chest.

Step 2: Quickly hop diagonally, shifting your weight onto the opposite leg. Bring the opposite arm up to your chest.

Step 3: Continue the movement, hopping on each leg diagonally forwards.

Tips: Perform a high leaping action. As a variation, you can reverse the movement.

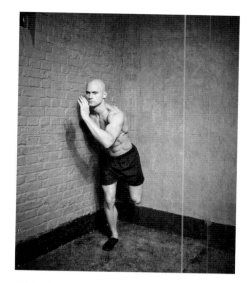

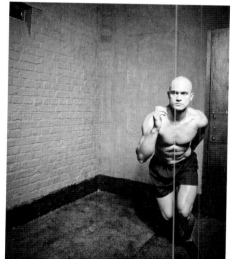

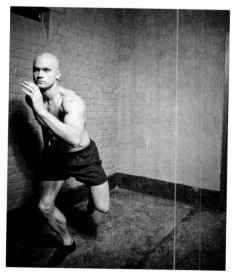

PLYO REVERSE TOUCHDOWN POWER SKIP

Target Muscle Groups

Primary: Quadriceps, Gluteals, Hamstrings

Secondary: Gastrocnemius, Soleus, Abdominals

Step 1: Step one leg back as far as you can into a reverse lunge and touch down with your hand. Take your other hand behind you. Keep your chest up and look ahead.

Step 2: Quickly bring your back leg forwards and up in line with your chest, whilst explosively pushing through your other leg to jump up as high as you can. At the same time, drive your opposite arm up and the other arm back with bent elbows to propel yourself upwards.

Step 3: Continue the movement, as you land on the same leg you pushed off with, decelerating with a soft knee. Return to the starting position. Repeat, then alternate sides.

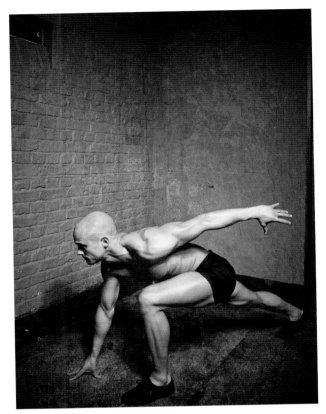

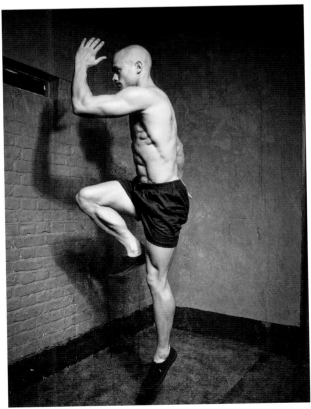

BURPEE

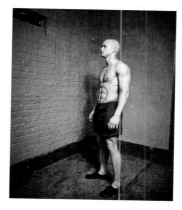

Target Muscle Groups
Primary: Quadriceps, Gluteals, Hamstrings
Secondary: Gastrocnemius, Soleus, Abdominals, Deltoids, Triceps

Step 1: Stand with feet shoulder-width apart and arms by your sides.

Step 2: Push your hips back, bend your knees and squat down as you place your hands on the floor in front of you, directly under your shoulders.

Step 3: Shift your weight onto your hands, then explosively, thrust your legs straight out behind you back into the press up position, toes tucked under and with your hands flat on the floor, arms straight.

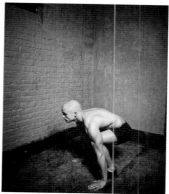

Step 4: Quickly jump your legs in so that your feet are under your chest, (as shown in the second image).

Step 5: Swing your arms to power up towards the ceiling while you jump up as high as possible.

Step 6: Continue the movement, decelerating with soft knees as you bend into a squat before returning to the upright standing position.

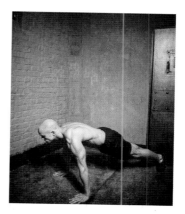

Tips: Do not let your lower back arch as you kick your legs back. Keep you abdominals engaged.

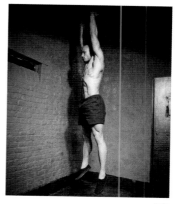

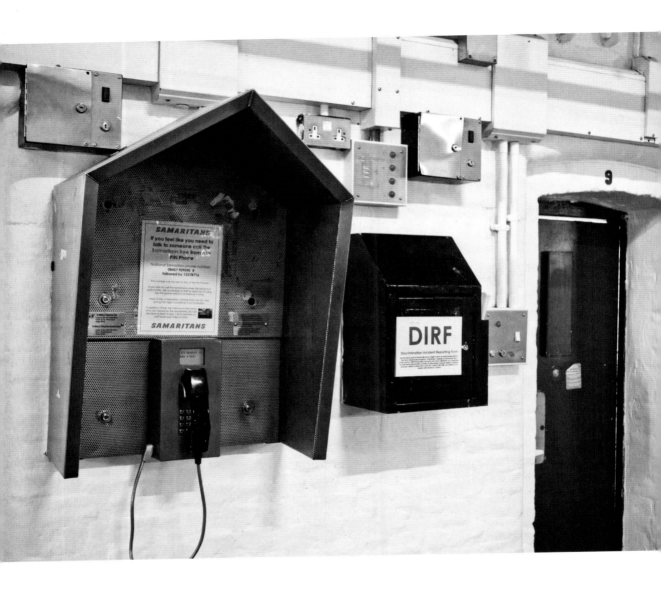

SHOULDERS

The function of the shoulders are to mobilise the upper limb, this involves the hand, forearm and arm. Primitively, this would have been useful for locomotion but in more recent times it allows us to reach out and grab or handle certain items.

It is a ball and socket joint involving numerous bones in the body; shoulder blade, upper arm and collar bone (the scapula, humerus and clavicle).

The shoulders can flex, extend and rotate the upper limb.

MUSCLE GROUPS

Deltoids
The deltoids are a large, triangular muscle, which forms the upper section of the arms. They can be divided further into three heads.

They originate from the lateral aspect of the clavicle, the superior part of the scapula and insert into the middle third of the humerus.

Basic function: the anterior deltoid raises the arm forwards (flex), the medial deltoid raises the arm out to the side (abduct) and the posterior deltoid extends the arm out behind the body (extension). When grouped together it allows us to rotate the upper limb and lift the arm.

Trapezius
The trapezius is a flat, triangular muscle, which extends from the neck down in between the shoulder blades.

The trapezius originates from the neck and thoracic spine. It then inserts into the spine of the scapula and outer third of the clavicle. When fully visualised this muscle covers a large portion of the back and extends to almost halfway down the spine.

Basic function: to lift the entire shoulder and upper limb, and help turn the head from side to side.

HAND PUSH

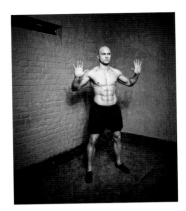

Target Muscle Groups
Primary: Deltoids, Pectorals
Secondary: Triceps, Abdominals

Step 1: Stand with your feet shoulder-width apart. Raise your hands out in front, at shoulder-height and held wider than your shoulders. Keep your arms slightly bent.

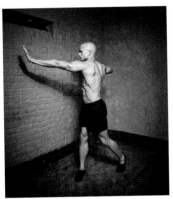

Step 2: Rotate at the hips and straighten one arm as you push your hand across your chest and out to the side, at shoulder-height. Lift up onto the toes of your back leg. This will help you reach further.

Step 3: Bring your hand back to return to the start position. Alternate on the other side.

SHOULDER PRESS WALL SLIDE

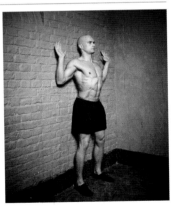

Target Muscle Groups
Primary: Deltoids
Secondary: Rhomboids, Trapezius, Triceps

Step 1: Stand with your back flat against the wall. Bend your elbows and raise your arms up, palms facing out, so that your hands are up in line with your ears.

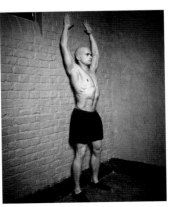

Step 2: Maintaining contact with the wall, press your arms back against the wall as you raise them up high.

Step 3: Lower your arms down to the starting position before pressing up again.

BENT ARM FRONT CROSS OVER

Target Muscle Groups
Primary: Deltoids
Secondary: Rhomboids, Trapezius

Step 1: Stand with your feet together. Bend your elbows and raise your arms up to shoulder-height, with your hands pointing forwards and palms facing down.

Step 2: Engage your core muscles and relax your shoulders. Slowly, bring the arms in towards each other so that one is held higher than the other in front of your chest.

Step 3: Slowly return your arms back to the start position.

Step 4: Repeat the action, bringing the arms in and out, alternating which arm is on top.

Tip: This exercise can be performed either standing or seated.

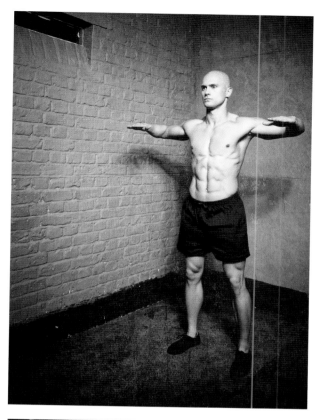

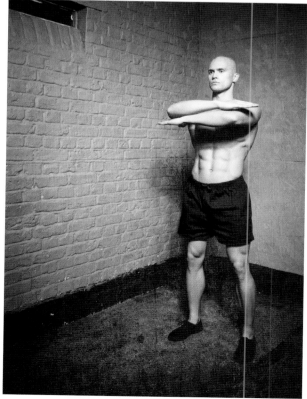

ELBOWS IN EXTERNAL ROTATION

Target Muscle Groups
Primary: Deltoids
Secondary:

Step 1: Stand with your feet hip-width apart. Bend your arms and tuck your elbows in tight by your sides, with your lower arms facing forwards. Clench your fists and keep your palms facing up.

Step 2: Keeping your elbows tucked in, rotate your hands outwards.

Step 3: Continue the movement, rotating your hands back to the start position.

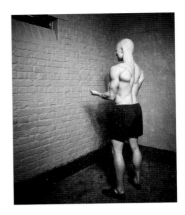

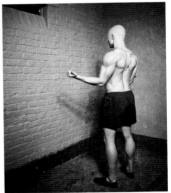

HAND GRASP PULL

Target Muscle Groups
Primary: Deltoids
Secondary: Triceps, Biceps

Step 1: Stand with your feet hip-width apart. Clasp your hands in front of your chest with your elbows bent and level with your shoulders.

Step 2: Keeping your hands clasped, pull against each other as if you are trying to separate them.

Step 3: Continue the movement, holding the tension and then release.

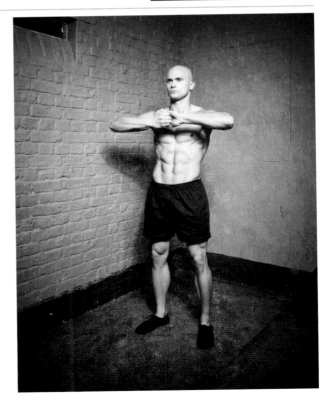

STANDING ARM DRIVE

Target Muscle Groups
Primary: Deltoids
Secondary: Triceps, Biceps, Abdominals

Step 1: Stand with one foot in front of the other. Bend your arms and keep your elbows by your sides.

Step 2: With hands open and arms bent, drive one elbow back and the other hand up, as in a running action, bringing your fingertips up to head height.

Step 3: Continue the movement, alternating your arms and gradually increase the speed.

Tip: This exercise can also be performed kneeling. With one knee touching the floor and the opposite foot positioned on the floor in front of you, in line with your ankle.

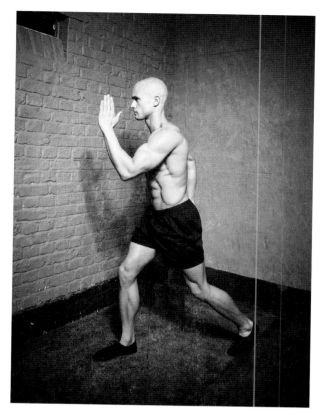

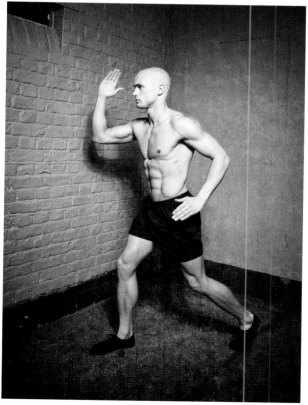

SUPINE SHOULDER FLEXION

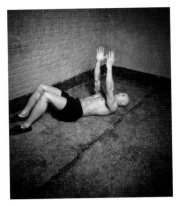

Target Muscle Groups
Primary: Deltoids
Secondary: Latissimus Dorsi

Step 1: Lie on your back, with your knees bent and feet flat on the floor, hip-width apart. Extend your arms straight up, fingers pointing towards the ceiling and palms facing inwards.

Step 2: Pull your shoulder blades down and maintain your lower back in contact with the floor. Keeping your arms straight, slowly lower both arms down onto the floor behind you.

Step 3: Continue the movement, slowly raising your arms back up to the start position.

Tip: This exercise can also be performed using alternate arms, lowering one down while holding the other still, pointing upwards.

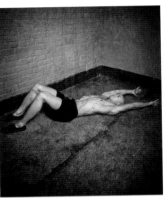

SUPINE SHOULDER LATERAL FLEXION

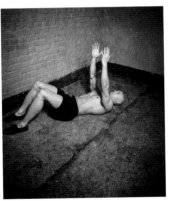

Target Muscle Groups
Primary: Deltoids, Pectorals
Secondary:

Step 1: Lie on your back, with your knees bent and feet flat on the floor, hip-width apart. Extend your arms straight up, fingers pointing towards the ceiling and palms facing inwards.

Step 2: Pull your shoulder blades down and maintain your lower back in contact with the floor. Slowly lower both arms out to the sides down onto the floor, keeping them level with your shoulders.

Step 3: Continue the movement, slowly raising your arms back up to the start position.

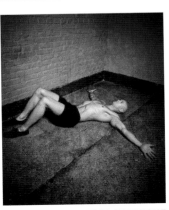

I FORMATION WITH ARMS IN FRONT

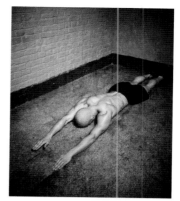

Target Muscle Groups
Primary: Deltoids
Secondary: Trapezius, Rhomboids

Step 1: Lie on your front with feet together and nose lightly touching the floor. Keep your head relaxed. Extend your arms straight up in front of your head, so that your body forms an 'I' formation.

Step 2: Looking down, keep your chest in contact with the floor and raise your arms off the ground, maintaining the 'I' formation.

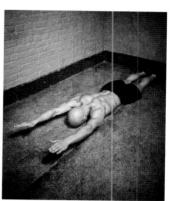

Step 3: Continue the movement, slowly lowering your arms back down to the start position.

Tip: This and the following formations can also be performed single arm.

Y FORMATION

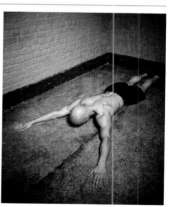

Target Muscle Groups
Primary: Deltoids
Secondary: Trapezius, Rhomboids

Step 1: Lie on your front with feet together and nose lightly touching the floor. Keep your head relaxed. Extend your arms up and outwards, until they are pointing 45-degrees above shoulder level, so that your arms and body form a 'Y' formation.

Step 2: Looking down, keep your chest in contact with the floor and raise your arms off the ground, maintaining the 'Y' formation.

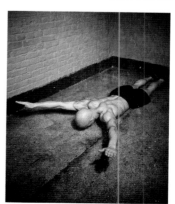

Step 3: Continue the movement, slowly lowering your arms back down to the start position.

T FORMATION

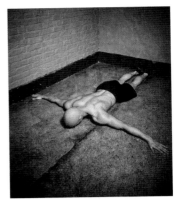

Target Muscle Groups
Primary: Deltoids
Secondary:

Step 1: Lie on your front with feet together and nose lightly touching the floor. Keep your head relaxed. Extend your arms straight out to the sides, in line with your shoulders, so that your arms and body form a 'T' formation.

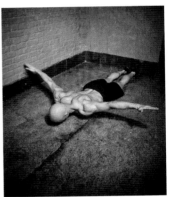

Step 2: Looking down, keep your chest in contact with the floor and raise your arms off the ground, maintaining the 'T' formation.

Step 3: Continue the movement, slowly lowering your arms back down to the start position.

L FORMATION

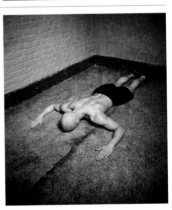

Target Muscle Groups
Primary: Deltoids, Pectorals
Secondary: Trapezius, Rhomboids

Step 1: Lie on your front with feet together and nose lightly touching the floor. Keep your head relaxed. With palms down, bend your elbows at 90-degrees so that your arms form two 'L' formations. Keep your elbows in line with your shoulders.

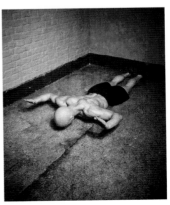

Step 2: Looking down, keep your chest in contact with the floor and raise your arms, maintaining the 'L' formation.

Step 3: Continue the movement, slowly lowering your arms back down to the start position.

W FORMATION

Target Muscle Groups
Primary: Deltoids
Secondary: Trapezius, Rhomboids

Step 1: Lie on your front with feet together and nose lightly touching the floor. Keep your head relaxed. With palms down, tuck your elbows in tight by your sides and move your arms so that your upper body forms a 'W' formation.

Step 2: Looking down, keep your chest in contact with the floor and raise your arms, maintaining the 'W' formation.

Step 3: Continue the movement, slowly lowering your arms back down to the start position.

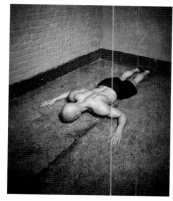

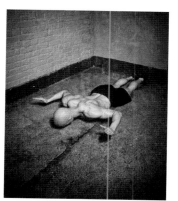

I FORMATION WITH ARMS BY SIDE

Target Muscle Groups
Primary: Deltoids
Secondary: Trapezius, Rhomboids, Triceps

Step 1: Lie on your front with feet together and nose lightly touching the floor. Keep your head relaxed. Extend your arms straight down by your sides, so that your body forms an 'I' formation.

Step 2: Looking down, keep your chest in contact with the floor and raise your arms, maintaining the 'I' formation.

Step 3: Continue the movement, slowly lowering your arms back down to the start position.

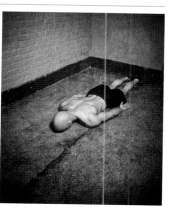

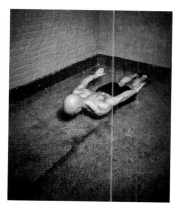

SUPINE SHOULDER ELEVATION

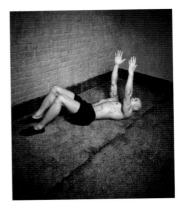

Target Muscle Groups
Primary: Deltoids
Secondary: Rhomboids, Trapezius

Step 1: Lie on your back, with your knees bent and feet flat on the floor, hip-width apart. With fingers pointed, extend your arms straight up in the air.

Step 2: Keeping your arms straight, slowly raise your arms up to lift your shoulder blades off the floor. Keep your lower back in contact with the floor.

Step 3: Continue the movement, slowly lowering your arms down, returning your shoulders to the start position.

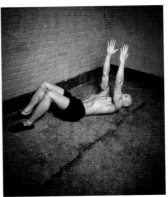

FAST HAND TAP

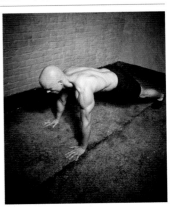

Target Muscle Groups
Primary: Deltoids
Secondary: Pectorals, Triceps

Step 1: Assume a standard full plank position, with your hands under your shoulders, feet hip-width apart and toes tucked under. Maintain a straight line from head to heels and look down at the floor.

Step 2: Engage your abdominals and keep your arms straight. Lift one hand and tap it down on top of your other hand.

Step 3: Continue the movement, returning back to the start position and alternating your hands. Gradually increase the speed.

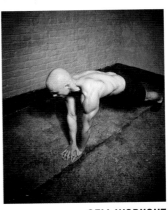

Tip: For an easier version, perform this exercise on your knees.

FULL PLANK BODYSAW

Target Muscle Groups
Primary: Deltoids, Abdominals
Secondary: Triceps

Step 1: Assume a standard full plank position, with your hands under your shoulders, feet hip-width apart and toes tucked under. Maintain a straight line from head to heels and look down at the floor.

Step 2: Engage your abdominals and keep your arms straight. Without moving your hands, raise up onto your toes pushing your body forward.

Step 3: Continue the movement, moving your body backwards to return to the start position.

Tip: Advanced variation; slowly rotate your shoulders and toes in a circular motion, maintaining a straight line from head to heels.

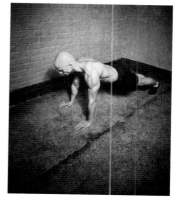

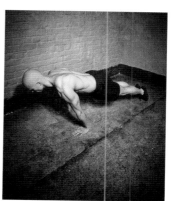

FULL PLANK BODYSAW WITH SINGLE LEG

Target Muscle Groups
Primary: Deltoids, Abdominals, Gluteals
Secondary: Triceps, Quadriceps

Step 1: Assume a standard full plank position, with your hands under your shoulders, feet hip-width apart and toes tucked under. Raise one foot off the floor, maintaining a straight line from head to heels and look down at the floor.

Step 2: Engage your abdominals and keep your arms straight. Without moving your hands, raise up onto your toes pushing your body forward.

Step 3: Continue the movement, moving your body backwards to return to the start position. Repeat, lifting the opposite leg.

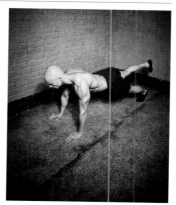

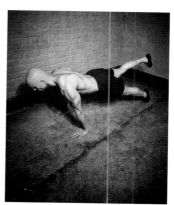

SIDE SINGLE ARM SHOULDER WALL PRESS

Target Muscle Groups
Primary: Deltoids
Secondary: Triceps

Step 1: Stand with feet together and a wall at arm's length to the side of you. Raise the arm closest to the wall up to shoulder height and gently press your palm and fingers onto the wall.

Step 2: Bend the supporting arm to lower your body towards the wall. Keep your body in a straight line.

Step 3: Continue the movement, pressing through your supporting arm to return your body back up to the upright start position. Repeat then alternate on the opposite side using the other arm.

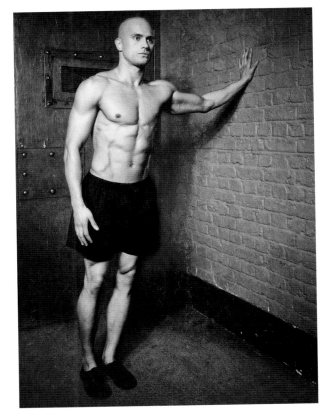

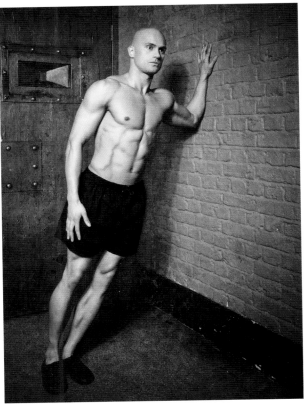

76

PIKE SHOULDER PRESS

Target Muscle Groups
Primary: Deltoids, Trapezius
Secondary: Triceps, Abdominals

Step 1: Assume a standard press up position, with arms straight, slightly wider than shoulder-width apart and with your feet hip-width apart and toes tucked under. Raise your hips up high and lift on to your toes to form a pike position.

Step 2: Maintaining the pike position with your body, bend your elbows outwards to lower your head to the floor.

Step 3: Continue the movement, pressing back up to return to start position.

Tip: To increase the difficulty of the exercise, walk your hands in towards your feet into a higher pike position.

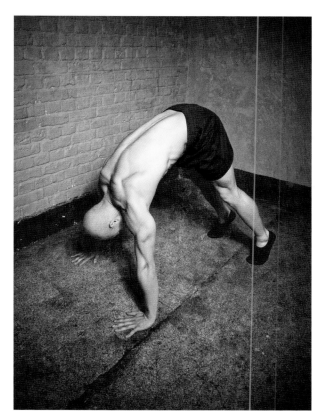

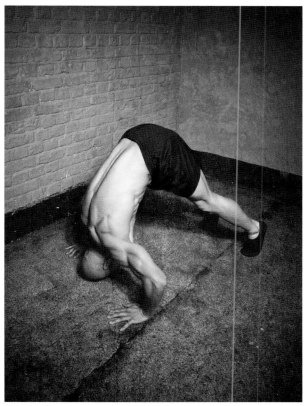

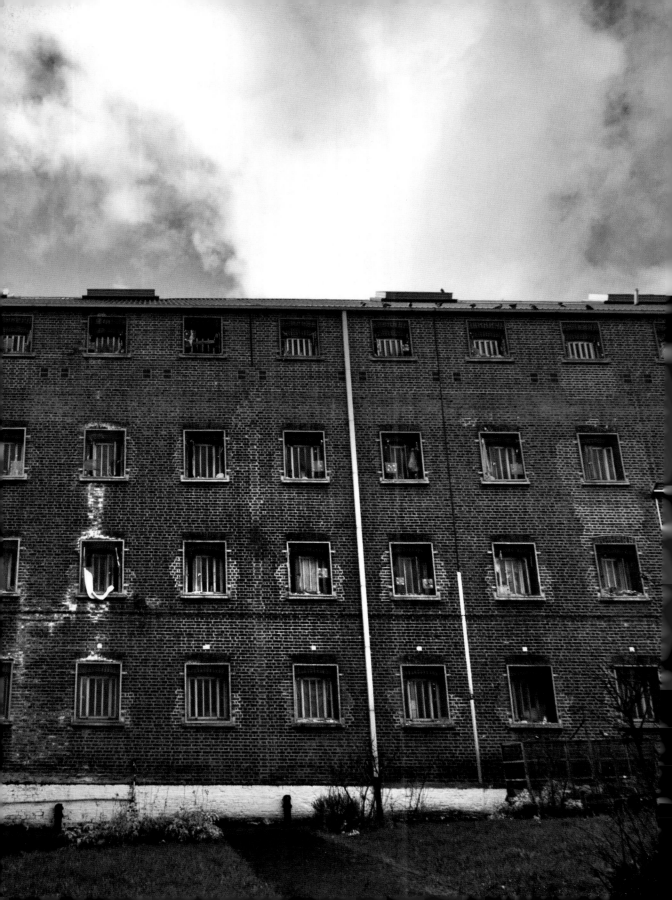

CHEST

The function of the chest is similar to that of the shoulders, to mobilise the upper limb. It covers a large area of the upper body and lies on top of the rib cage.

When the chest becomes well developed it gives an impressive appearance that many aspire to.

MUSCLE GROUPS

Pectorals (Pecs)
The pectorals, commonly known as 'pecs' are made up of two muscles; the pectoralis major and pectoralis minor.

Major
The pectoralis major originates from the sternum and middle portion of the collar bone (clavicle), it spreads outwards and fans across the body where it attaches to the upper portion of the arm (humerus).

Minor
The pectoralis minor lies underneath the pectoralis major and is a thin triangular muscle. It originates from the upper ribs and attaches to the underside of the shoulder blade (scapula).

When the two muscles are grouped together they work to produce the same function.

Basic function: *to pull the arm and shoulder across the front of the body.*

WALL PRESS UP

Target Muscle Groups
Primary: Pectorals
Secondary: Triceps, Deltoids

Step 1: Stand facing a wall, feet hip-width apart. Place your hands on the wall, wider than shoulder-width apart and level with your shoulders. Position your feet at a distance from the wall so that you are leaning slightly forwards and your arms have a slight bend at the elbow.

Step 2: Bend your elbows and lower yourself towards the wall until your nose nearly touches the wall.

Step 3: Continue the movement, pressing back out to the start position.

Tip: The further you stand from the wall the more challenging the exercise will be.

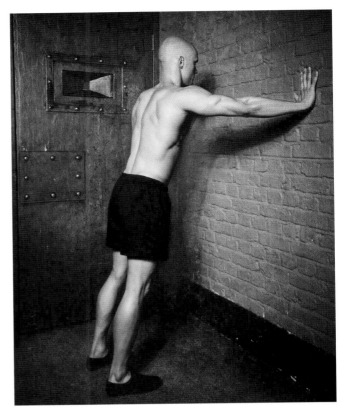

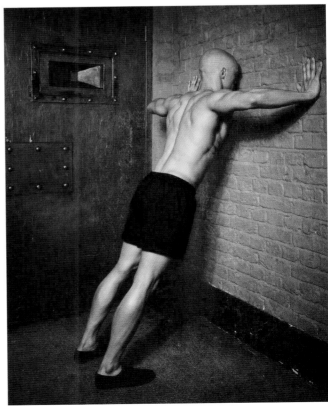

CLOSE HAND WALL PRESS UP

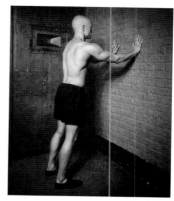

Target Muscle Groups
Primary: Pectorals, Triceps
Secondary: Deltoids

Step 1: Stand facing a wall, feet hip-width apart.
Place your hands on the wall, shoulder-width apart
and inline with your shoulders. Position your feet
at a distance from the wall so that you are leaning
slightly forwards and your arms have a slight bend
at the elbow.

Step 2: Bend your elbows and lower yourself
towards the wall until your nose nearly touches the
wall. Keep your elbows tucked into your sides.

Step 3: Continue the movement, pressing back out to
the start position.

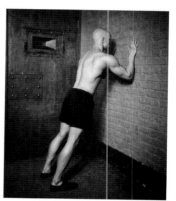

SINGLE ARM WALL PRESS UP

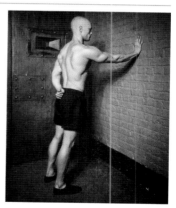

Target Muscle Groups
Primary: Pectorals
Secondary: Triceps, Deltoids, Abdominals

Step 1: Stand facing a wall, feet hip-width apart.
Place one hand on the wall, in line with your
shoulder and the other behind your back. Position
your feet at a distance from the wall so that you are
leaning slightly forwards and your arm has a slight
bend at the elbow.

Step 2: Bend your elbow and lower yourself towards
the wall until your nose nearly touches the wall.

Step 3: Continue the movement, pressing back out
to the start position. Repeat, then alternate using the
opposite arm.

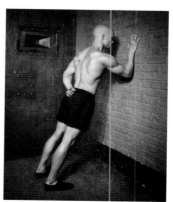

PRESS UP ON KNEES

Target Muscle Groups
Primary: Pectorals
Secondary: Triceps, Deltoids

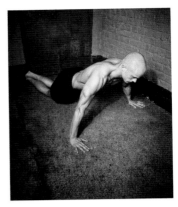

Step 1: Kneel on all fours, with your hands slightly wider than shoulder-width apart, fingers facing forwards and spread wide. Your knees should be hip-width apart and bent slightly behind your hips.

Step 2: With eyes looking down, slowly bend your elbows and point them outwards as you lower your body towards the floor. Keep your body in a straight line throughout the movement.

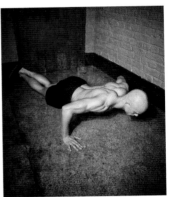

Step 3: Continue the movement, pressing through your hands, straightening your elbows, to return to the start position.

CLOSE HAND PRESS UP ON KNEES

Target Muscle Groups
Primary: Pectorals
Secondary: Triceps, Deltoids

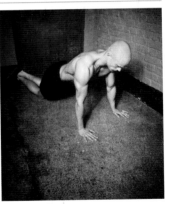

Step 1: Kneel on all fours, with your hands directly under your shoulders, fingers facing forwards and spread wide. Your knees should be hip-width apart and bent slightly behind your hips.

Step 2: With eyes looking down, slowly bend your elbows and tuck them in by your sides, as you lower your body towards the floor. Keep your body in a straight line throughout the movement.

Step 3: Continue the movement, pressing through your hands, straightening your elbows, to return to the start position.

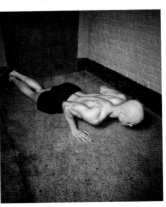

PRESS UP

Target Muscle Groups
Primary: Pectorals
Secondary: Triceps, Deltoids

Step 1: Start on the floor in a downward facing position, with your hands placed slightly wider than shoulder-width apart, fingers facing forwards and spread wide. Extend your legs straight behind you with your feet at hip-width apart, toes tucked under.

Step 2: With eyes looking down, slowly bend your elbows, pointing them outwards, as you lower your body towards the floor. Keep your body in a straight line throughout the movement.

Step 3: Continue the movement, pressing through your hands, straightening your elbows, to return to the start position.

Tip: To make the exercise harder place your feet closer together, to make it easier place them wider than hip-width.

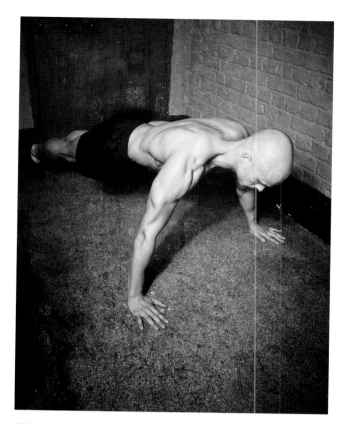

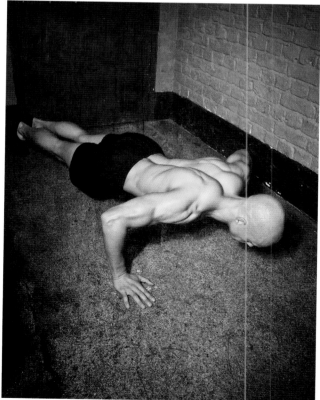

WIDE HAND PRESS UP

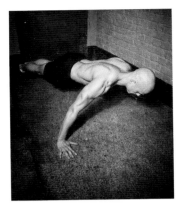

Target Muscle Groups
Primary: Pectorals
Secondary: Triceps, Deltoids

Step 1: Assume a standard press up position. Walk each hand out wider than shoulder-width apart. Engage your abdominals, keep your head and neck aligned with your spine and your body in a straight line.

Step 2: With eyes looking down, slowly bend your elbows, pointing them outwards, as you lower your body towards the floor. Keep your body in a straight line throughout the movement.

Step 3: Continue the movement, pressing through your hands, straightening your elbows, to return to the start position.

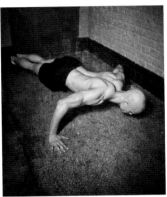

CLOSE HAND PRESS UP

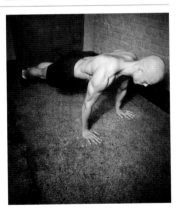

Target Muscle Groups
Primary: Pectorals, Triceps
Secondary: Deltoids

Step 1: Assume a standard press up position. Walk your hands in so they are directly under your shoulders. Engage your abdominals, keep your head and neck aligned with your spine and your body in a straight line.

Step 2: Slowly bend your elbows, keeping them tucked in by your sides and lower your body towards the floor. Keep your body in a straight line throughout the movement.

Step 3: Continue the movement, pressing through your hands, straightening your elbows, to return to the start position.

Tip: This exercise will place more emphasis on the triceps than a standard press up.

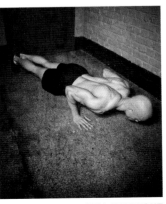

DIAMOND PRESS UP

Target Muscle Groups
Primary: Pectorals, Triceps
Secondary: Deltoids

Step 1: Assume a standard press up position. Place your hands together to form a diamond shape with your fingers and thumbs, directly under your chest.

Step 2: With eyes looking down, slowly bend your elbows with your chest directly over your hands and elbows tucked in by your sides.

Step 3: Continue the movement, pressing through your hands, straightening your elbows, to return to the start position.

Tips: When performing the various press ups, with your hands wider apart, the distance of movement will lessen from the standard press up. When closer together the distance will increase.

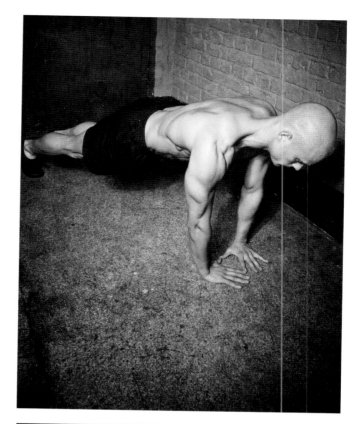

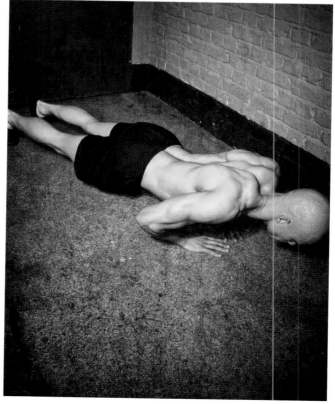

CHEST

STACKED FEET PRESS UP

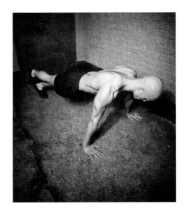

Target Muscle Groups
Primary: Pectorals
Secondary: Triceps, Deltoids, Abdominals

Step 1: Assume a standard press up position. Place one foot directly on top of the other. Engage your abdominals and maintain your body in a straight line.

Step 2: With eyes looking down, slowly bend your elbows, pointing them outwards, as you lower your body towards the floor. Keep your body in a straight line throughout the movement.

Step 3: Continue the movement, pressing through your hands, straightening your elbows, to return to the start position. Repeat, stacking the opposite foot on top.

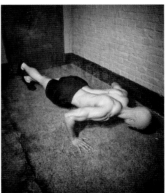

STAGGERED HAND PRESS UP

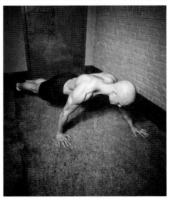

Target Muscle Groups
Primary: Pectorals
Secondary: Triceps, Deltoids

Step 1: Assume a standard press up position. Place your hands facing forwards, one slightly in front and one slightly behind your shoulders and both feet together directly behind you. Engage your abdominals and maintain your body in a straight line.

Step 2: With eyes looking down, slowly bend your elbows, pointing them outwards, as you lower your body towards the floor.

Step 3: Continue the movement, pressing through your hands, straightening your elbows, to return to the start position. Repeat, alternating sides, varying hand positions accordingly.

Tip: As you progress with this exercise, improvise with your hand placement.

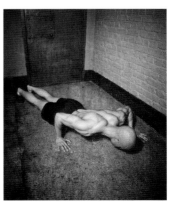

FRONT LOADED PRESS UP

Target Muscle Groups
Primary: Pectorals
Secondary: Triceps, Deltoids

Step 1: Assume a standard press up position with your elbows tucked into your sides. Engage your abdominals and maintain your body in a straight line.

Step 2: With eyes looking down, slowly bend your elbows, keeping them tucked in by your sides, as you lower your body towards the floor.

Step 3: Roll from the balls of your feet onto your toes, moving your body forwards until your shoulders are in front of your hands. Maintain your body in a straight line throughout the exercise.

Step 4: Continue the movement, rolling back onto the balls of your feet. Press through your hands, straightening your elbows to return to the start position.

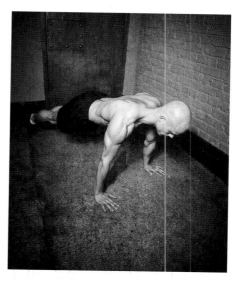

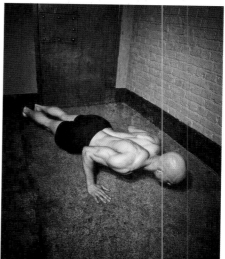

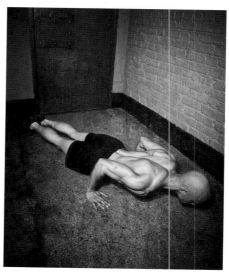

LATERAL PRESS UP

Target Muscle Groups
Primary: Pectorals
Secondary: Triceps, Deltoids, Abdominals

Step 1: Assume a standard press up position. Engage your abdominals and maintain your body in a straight line.

Step 2: With eyes looking down, slowly bend your elbows, pointing them outwards, as you lower your body towards the floor.

Step 3: Press through your hands as you straighten your elbows, walk one hand inwards placing it next to the opposite hand, positioning your hands directly under your chest

Step 4: Continue the movement, walking the stationary hand outwards, until they are shoulder-width apart. Repeat, alternating the direction.

Tip: Try moving in a full circle then reversing in the opposite direction.

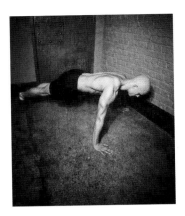

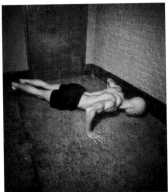

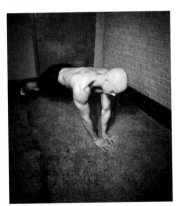

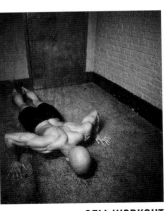

CHEST SQUEEZE

Target Muscle Groups
Primary: Pectorals
Secondary: Deltoids, Triceps, Biceps

Step 1: Stand with feet hip-width apart. Bend your arms in front of your chest, keeping elbows wide, and place the palms of your hands together with fingers facing upwards.

Step 2: Press both hands against each other increasing the tension as you contract your chest. Keep your breathing normal throughout.

Step 3: Continue the movement, holding the tension for the desired length of time. Release the tension slowly.

Tips: You can perform this exercise by changing the angle of the hands, above or below parallel. Or place a hard object, such as a book, in between your hands.

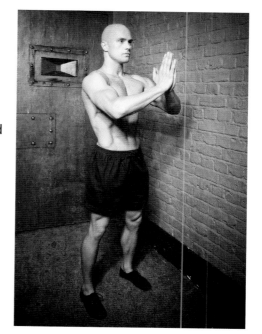

STRAIGHT ARM CHEST SQUEEZE

Target Muscle Groups
Primary: Pectorals
Secondary: Deltoids, Triceps, Biceps

Step 1: Stand with feet hip-width apart. Extend your arms straight out in front of your chest, at shoulder-height and place the palms of your hands together, with fingers pointing forwards.

Step 2: Press both hands against each other increasing the tension as you contract your chest. Keep your breathing normal throughout.

Step 3: Continue the movement, holding the tension for the desired length of time. Release the tension slowly.

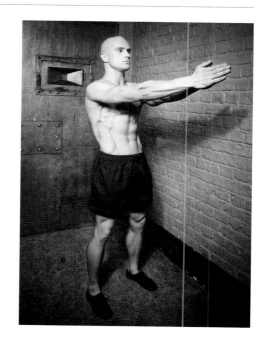

PRAYING HAND RAISE WITH CHEST SQUEEZE

Target Muscle Groups
Primary: Pectorals
Secondary: Deltoids, Triceps, Biceps

Step 1: Stand with feet hip-width apart. Bend your elbows to a 90-degree angle and touch them together at shoulder-height. Keep your palms together and fingers pointing up.

Step 2: Squeeze your elbows, forearms and palms together. Raise your hands upwards as you contract your chest.

Step 3: Continue the movement, lowering your arms down to the start position. Release the tension slowly.

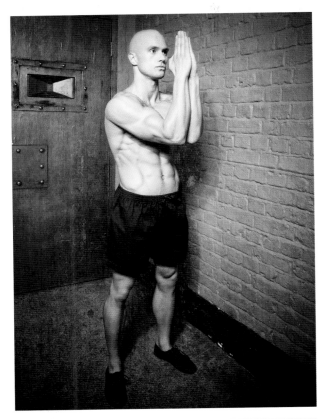

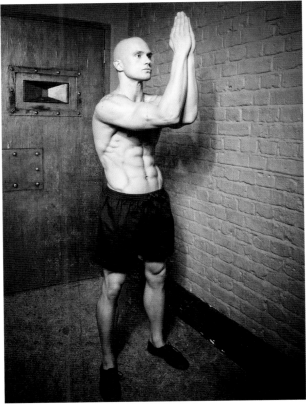

PLYO PRESS UP

Target Muscle Groups
Primary: Pectorals
Secondary: Triceps, Deltoids, Abdominals

Step 1: Assume a standard press up position. Engage your abdominals and maintain your body in a straight line.

Step 2: With eyes looking down, slowly bend your elbows, pointing them outwards, as you lower your body towards the floor. Keep your body in a straight line throughout the movement.

Step 3: Continue the movement, explosively pressing up with enough force so that your hands come up off the floor. As your hands touch back down onto the floor, decelerate to lower your body down in a controlled movement.

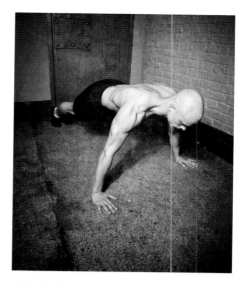

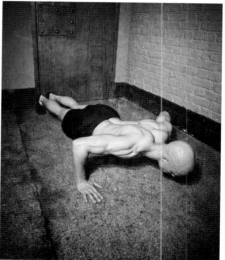

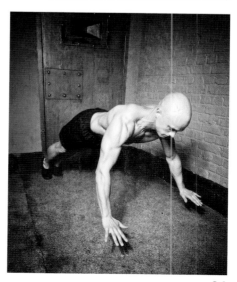

PLYO STAGGERED HAND PRESS UP

Target Muscle Groups
Primary: Pectorals
Secondary: Triceps, Deltoids, Abdominals

Step 1: Assume a standard press up position. Place your hands facing forwards, one slightly in front and one slightly behind your shoulders and both feet together directly behind you.

Step 2: With eyes looking down, slowly bend your elbows, pointing them outwards, as you lower your body towards the floor. Keep your body in a straight line throughout the movement.

Step 3: Continue the movement, explosively pressing up with enough force so that your hands come up off the floor. Switch your hand positions mid-air, landing with the opposite hand in front.

Step 4: As your hands touch back down onto the floor, decelerate to lower your body down in a controlled movement. Repeat, alternating the hand positions as they land.

Tip: Improvise with your hand placement.

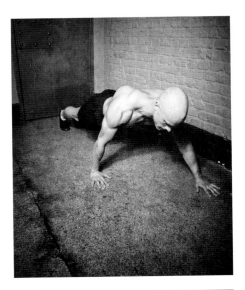

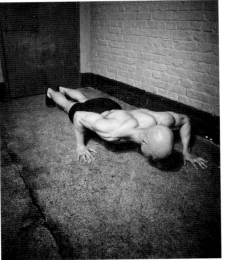

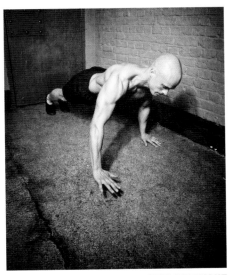

PLYO LATERAL PRESS UP

Target Muscle Groups
Primary: Pectorals
Secondary: Triceps, Deltoids, Abdominals

Step 1: Assume a standard press up position. Engage your abdominals and maintain your body in a straight line.

Step 2: With eyes looking down, slowly bend your elbows, pointing them outwards, as you lower your body towards the floor. Keep your body in a straight line throughout the movement.

Step 3: Continue the movement, explosively pressing up with enough force so that your hands come up off the floor moving your body over to one side mid-air, with your feet remaining on the floor.

Step 4: As your hands touch back down onto the floor, decelerate to lower your body down in a controlled movement. Repeat, alternating sides.

Tip: Try travelling round in one direction then reverse to travel back.

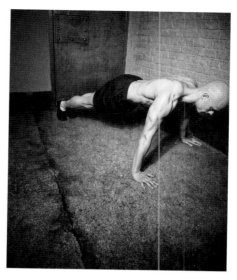

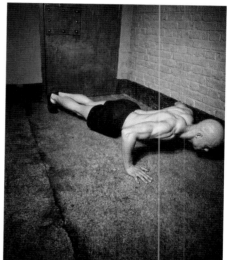

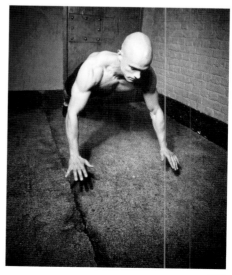

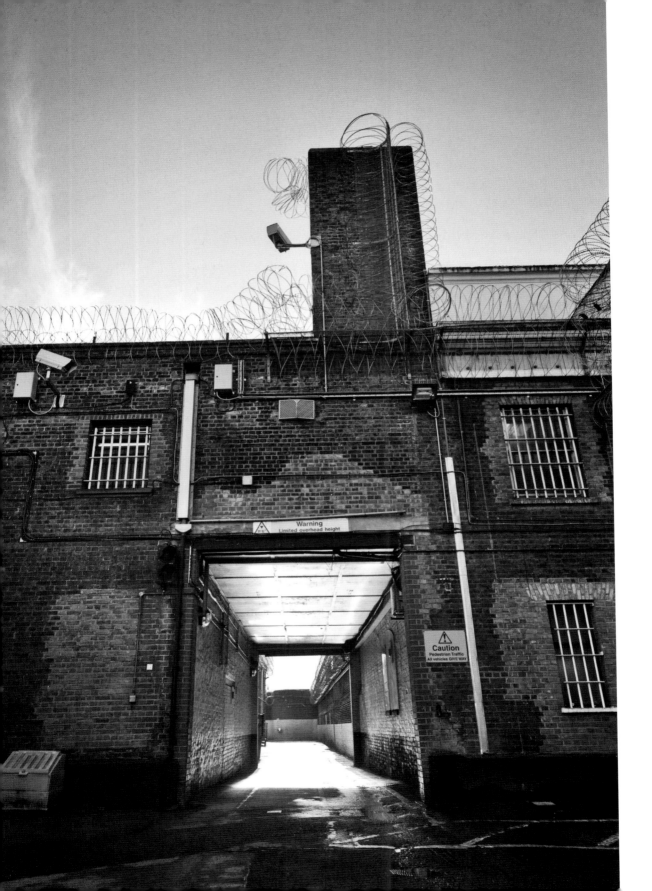

BACK

The back runs all the way from the neck to the top of the glutes. There are many muscles in the back and it is an incredibly strong part of the body.

These muscles are important for posture, support and flexibility.

The back doesn't, as such, have a joint movement itself, but allows for flexion, extension, lateral flexion and rotation of the spine.

MUSCLE GROUPS

Latissimus Dorsi

The latissimus dorsi or more commonly known as the 'lats', are the largest muscles of the upper body. They originate from the hip and lower portion of the spine and fan out over the shoulder blades (scapulae) and attach to the back of the upper arm (humerus) creating a triangular shape.

Basic function: *to pull the shoulders downwards and assist in bending the body from side to side.*

Rhomboids

The rhomboids, like the pecs, have a major and minor. They are located underneath the trapezius muscle and are rhombus shaped. They originate from the upper portion of the spine and attach to the shoulder blade (scapula).

Basic function: *to retract the shoulder blades (scapulae).*

Erector Spinae

The erector spinae are a group of muscles in the back (iliocostalis, longissimus, spinalis), which originate from the back of the rib cage and attach to the spine. They guard the nerves that supply the spinal cord. They are also the slowest muscles to recover once they have been fatigued through exercise.

Basic function: *to support the spinal column.*

GOOD MORNING

Target Muscle Groups
Primary: Erector Spinae
Secondary: Gluteals, Hamstrings

Step 1: Stand with your feet hip-width apart. Place your hands on your hips. Engage your abdominals, keep your neck aligned with your spine and look straight ahead.

Step 2: With a slight bend in your knees, bend forwards from the hips and lower your upper body until it is parallel to the floor.

Step 3: Continue the movement, slowly raising your upper body back to the start position.

Tip: To make the exercise harder place your feet closer together, to make it easier place them wider than hip-width.

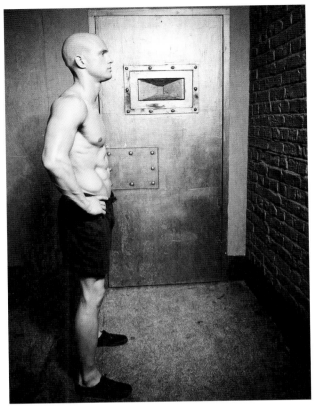

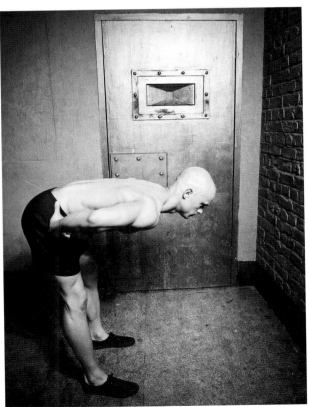

GOOD MORNING WITH ARMS BY SIDE

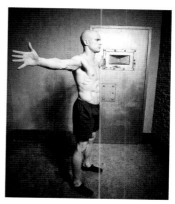

Target Muscle Groups
Primary: Erector Spinae, Rhomboids
Secondary: Gluteus, Hamstrings

Step 1: Stand with your feet hip-width apart. Extend your arms straight out to the side at shoulder height. Engage your abdominals, keep your neck aligned with your spine and look straight ahead.

Step 2: With a slight bend in your knees, bend forwards from the hips and lower your upper body until it is parallel to the floor.

Step 3: Continue the movement, slowly raising your upper body back to the start position.

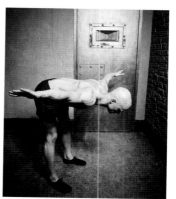

GOOD MORNING WITH ARMS ABOVE

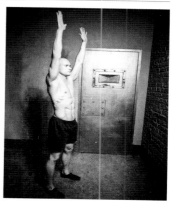

Target Muscle Groups
Primary: Erector Spinae, Rhomboids
Secondary: Gluteus, Hamstrings

Step 1: Stand with your feet hip-width apart. Extend your arms straight up above your head. Engage your abdominals, keep your neck aligned with your spine and look straight ahead.

Step 2: With a slight bend in your knees, bend forwards from the hips and lower your upper body until it is parallel to the floor.

Step 3: Continue the movement, slowly raising your upper body back to the start position.

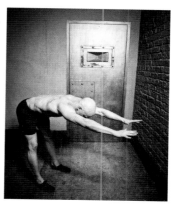

CAT COW

Target Muscle Groups
Primary: Erector Spinae, Rhomboids
Secondary: Abdominals

Step 1: Kneel on all fours, with a flat back, your hands directly under your shoulders and a slight bend in your elbows. Position your knees directly under your hips.

Step 2: Engage your abdominals. Lift your head, extend your neck forwards and arch your lower back into a stretch.

Step 3: Continue the movement, lowering your head whilst raising your upper back. Round your spine as you curl your tailbone under. Slowly return to the start position.

Tip: This exercise will strengthen your back and prevent back pain.

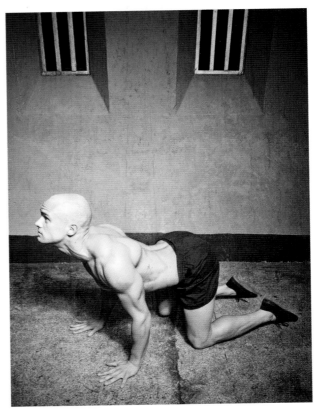

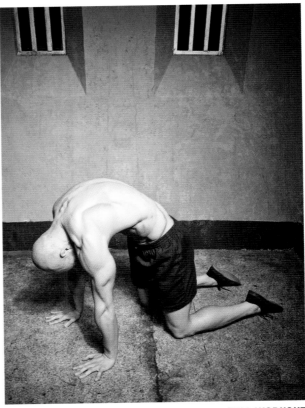

CHILDS POSE WITH ARM SWEEP

Target Muscle Groups
Primary: Deltoids, Erector Spinae, Latissimus Dorsi
Secondary: Gluteus, Rhomboids, Trapezius

Step 1: Kneel on all fours. Lower your hips back to sit on your heels, resting your chest on your thighs and round your spine. Stretch your arms out in front and lower your head on the floor.

Step 2: Slowly sweep your arms round so that your hands are by your feet.

Step 3: Continue the movement, sweeping your arms back to the start position.

Tip: This exercise can be performed stationary with your arms stretched out in front or by your feet.

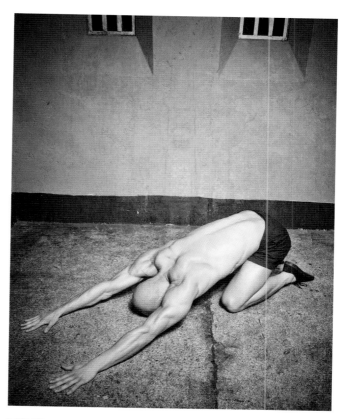

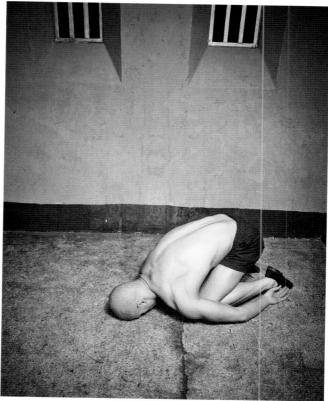

BABY COBRA

Target Muscle Groups
Primary: Erector Spinae, Rhomboids
Secondary: Triceps, Abdominals

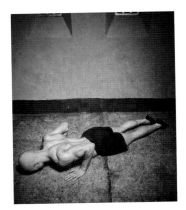

Step 1: Lie on your front, with hands positioned by your chest and fingers facing forwards, palms flat on the floor. Maintain straight legs and keep your toes pointed. Engage your abdominals.

Step 2: Focus your eyes down as you push down through your arms to slowly raise your upper body halfway up, so that your elbows are bent. Keep your hips and lower body fixed on the floor.

Step 3: Continue the movement, slowly lowering back down to the floor, lengthening the spine.

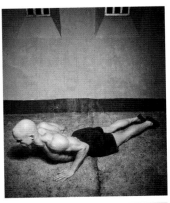

Tip: Use the support of your arms to help with lifting motion. As you become stronger, focus on using your lower back muscles to perform the raise, instead of your arms.

COBRA

Target Muscle Groups
Primary: Erector Spinae, Rhomboids
Secondary: Triceps, Abdominals

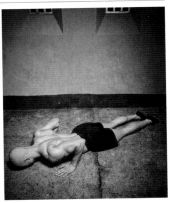

Step 1: Lie on your front, with hands positioned by your chest and fingers facing forwards, palms flat on the floor. Maintain straight legs and keep your toes pointed. Engage your abdominals.

Step 2: Focus your eyes down as you push down through your arms to slowly raise your upper body until your arms are almost straight. Keep your hips and lower body fixed on the floor.

Step 3: Continue the movement, slowly lowering back down to the floor, lengthening the spine.

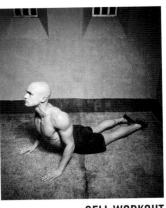

CELL WORKOUT

DOWN DOG UP DOG

Target Muscle Groups

Primary: Erector Spinae, Abdominals, Rhomboids, Gluteals

Secondary: Triceps, Deltoids, Hamstrings, Gastrocnemius

Step 1: Assume a standard press up position, with your hands shoulder-width apart. Push your hips up and backwards, bringing your chest towards thighs. Straighten your legs and flatten your heels to the floor. Relax your head between your shoulders.

Step 2: Lower your body, bending your arms, keeping elbows close to your sides.

Step 3: Push through your arms, lifting your body up and forwards, coming onto your toes. Raise your head and chest to look upwards, stretching your neck and arching your lower back.

Step 4: Continue the movement, bending your elbows, lowering your upper body and pushing your hips up and backwards to the start position.

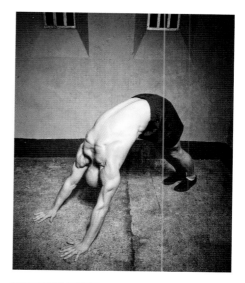

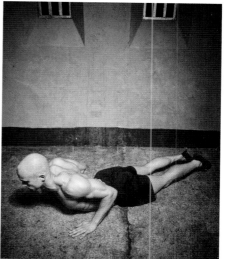

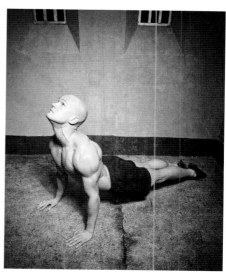

BACK

DORSAL RAISE WITH FINGERS ON TEMPLES

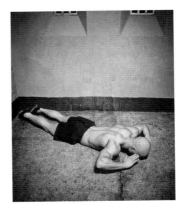

Target Muscle Groups
Primary: Erector Spinae, Rhomboids
Secondary:

Step 1: Lie on your front, with your legs extended straight behind you. Place your hands by your temples, elbows out wide. Keep your eyes fixed on the floor and your neck and head in a neutral position. Engage your abdominals.

Step 2: Slowly raise your head and chest off the floor, maintaining contact with your hips on the floor.

Step 3: Continue the movement, slowly lowering your chest back down to the start position.

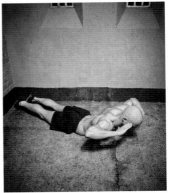

DORSAL RAISE WITH ROTATION

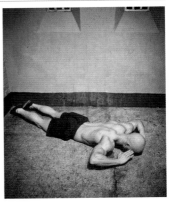

Target Muscle Groups
Primary: Erector Spinae, Rhomboids
Secondary: Obliques

Step 1: Lie on your front, with your legs extended straight behind you. Place your hands by your temples, elbows out wide. Keep your eyes fixed on the floor and your neck and head in a neutral position. Engage your abdominals.

Step 2: Slowly raise your head and chest off the floor, maintaining contact with your hips on the floor. Rotate your upper body to one side.

Step 3: Continue the movement, returning back to the center position and slowly lowering your chest back down to the start position. Repeat, rotating to the other side.

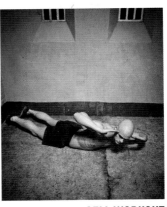

DORSAL RAISE WITH SIDE BEND

Target Muscle Groups
Primary: Erector Spinae, Rhomboids
Secondary: Obliques

Step 1: Lie on your front, with your legs extended straight behind you. Place your hands down by your sides. Keep your eyes fixed on the floor and your neck and head in a neutral position. Engage your abdominals.

Step 2: Slowly raise your head and chest off the floor, maintaining contact with your hips on the floor. Bend at the hips to reach down to one side.

Step 3: Continue the movement, returning back to the center position and slowly lower your chest back down to the start position. Repeat, bending to the other side.

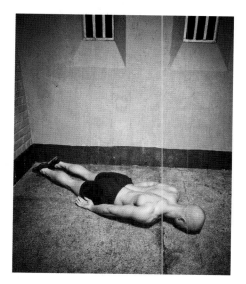

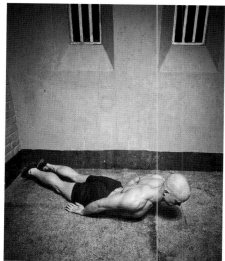

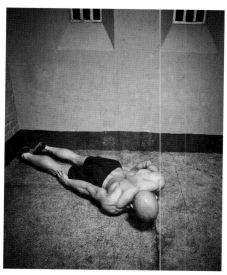

DORSAL RAISE WITH HANDS CLASPED BEHIND BACK

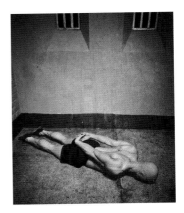

Target Muscle Groups
Primary: Erector Spinae, Rhomboids
Secondary: Deltoids, Trapezius, Triceps

Step 1: Lie on your front, with your legs extended straight behind you. Place your arms behind your back, with your hands clasped.

Step 2: Engage your abdominals. Slowly raise your arms, head and chest off the floor, maintaining contact with your hips on the floor.

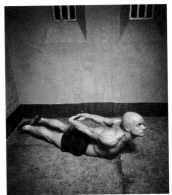

Step 3: Continue the movement, slowly lowering your chest and arms back down to the start position.

FINGER TIP ROTATION

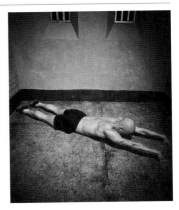

Target Muscle Groups
Primary: Erector Spinae, Rhomboids, Deltoids
Secondary: Obliques

Step 1: Lie on your front, with your legs extended straight behind you and your arms extended straight in front, raised on fingertips. Engage your abdominals and keep your neck and head in a neutral position.

Step 2: Slowly raise your head and chest off the floor, maintaining contact with your hips on the floor. Rotating at the hips, raise one arm and reach round and back opening your chest. Turn your head round to look up at your outstretched hand.

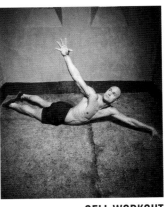

Step 3: Continue the movement, slowly returning your arm and chest back to the start position. Repeat, alternating on the other side.

BLACKBURN

Target Muscle Groups
Primary: Erector Spinae, Rhomboids, Latissimus Dorsi
Secondary: Deltoids

Step 1: Lie on your front, with your legs extended straight behind you and your arms extended straight in front. Keep your eyes fixed on the floor and your neck and head in a neutral position. Engage your abdominals.

Step 2: Slowly raise your arms, head and chest off the floor, maintaining contact with your hips on the floor. Keeping your arms straight, sweep your hands round until they are by your sides.

Step 3: Continue the movement, sweeping your arms back round above your head. Slowly lower your chest and arms back down to the start position.

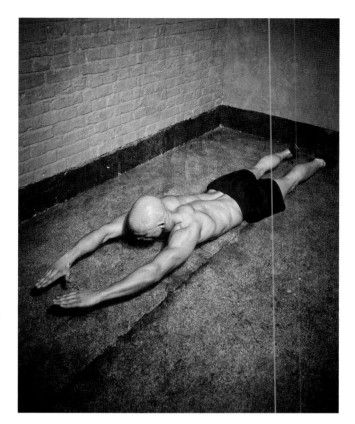

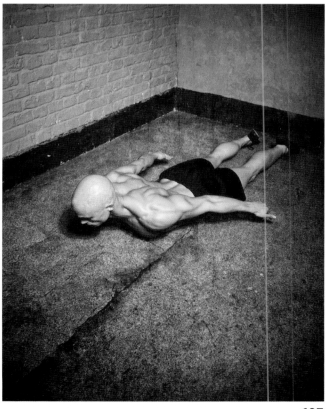

BACK PULL

Target Muscle Groups
Primary: Erector Spinae, Rhomboids, Latissimus Dorsi
Secondary: Deltoids

Step 1: Lie on your front, with your legs extended straight behind you and your arms extended straight in front. Engage your abdominals and keep your neck and head in a neutral position.

Step 2: Slowly raise your arms, head and chest off the floor, maintaining contact with your hips on the floor. Bend your elbows and pull your arms down, pulling your shoulders back and down.

Step 3: Continue the movement, releasing your arms and extend them to back above your head. Slowly lower your chest and arms back down to the start position.

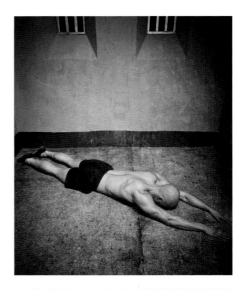

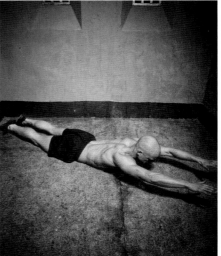

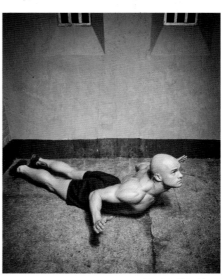

REVERSE DORSAL RAISE WITH SINGLE LEG

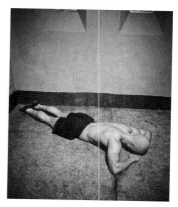

Target Muscle Groups
Primary: Erector Spinae, Gluteals
Secondary: Hamstrings

Step 1: Lie on your front, with your legs extended behind you and feet together. Place your hands directly under your head and palms flat on the floor. Rest your head on your hands.

Step 2: With your upper body in contact with the floor, slowly raise one leg up behind you, keeping the leg straight.

Step 3: Continue the movement, slowly lowering your leg back down to the start position. Repeat, alternating using the opposite leg.

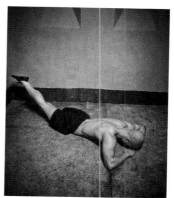

BACK

REVERSE DORSAL RAISE WITH DOUBLE LEG

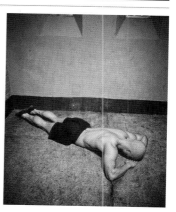

Target Muscle Groups
Primary: Erector Spinae, Gluteals
Secondary: Hamstrings

Step 1: Lie on your front, with your legs extended behind you and feet together. Place your hands directly under your head and palms flat on the floor. Rest your head on your hands.

Step 2: With your upper body in contact with the floor, slowly raise both legs up behind you, keeping the legs straight.

Step 3: Continue the movement, slowly lowering your legs back down to the start position.

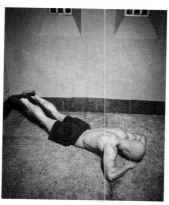

PRONE HEEL RAISE WITH SINGLE LEG

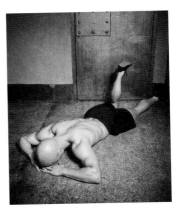

Target Muscle Groups
Primary: Erector Spinae, Gluteals
Secondary: Hamstrings

Step 1: Lie on your front, with one leg extended behind you and bend the other leg at 90-degrees. Place your hands directly under your head and palms flat on the floor. Rest your head on your hands.

Step 2: Lift the heel of your bent leg up towards the ceiling so that your thigh raises off the floor, keeping your upper body in contact with the floor.

Step 3: Continue the movement, lowering your leg back down to the start position. Repeat, raising the opposite leg.

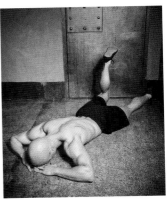

PRONE HEEL RAISE WITH DOUBLE LEG

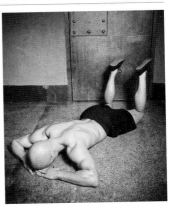

Target Muscle Groups
Primary: Erector Spinae, Gluteals
Secondary: Hamstrings

Step 1: Lie on your front, bending both knees at 90-degrees behind you. Place your hands directly under your head and palms flat on the floor. Rest your head on your hands.

Step 2: Lift your heels up towards the ceiling so that your thighs raise off the floor, keeping your upper body in contact with the floor.

Step 3: Continue the movement, lowering your thighs back down to the start position.

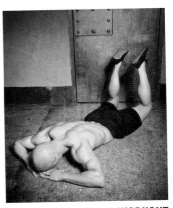

PRONE SCISSORS

Target Muscle Groups
Primary: Erector Spinae, Gluteals
Secondary: Hamstrings

Step 1: Lie on your front, with your legs extended behind you and feet together. Place your hands directly under your head and palms flat on the floor. Rest your head on your hands.

Step 2: With your upper body in contact with the floor, slowly raise both legs up behind you, keeping the legs straight. Cross the feet one over the other.

Step 3: Continue the movement, alternating the other foot on top, in a scissor action.

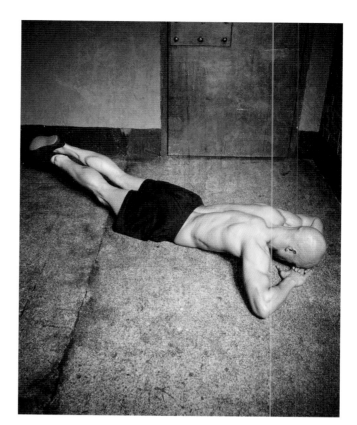

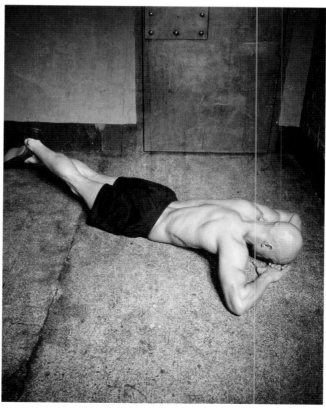

FULL DORSAL RAISE WITH ARMS BY SIDE

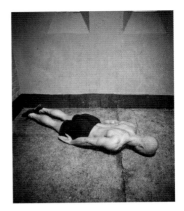

Target Muscle Groups
Primary: Erector Spinae, Gluteals, Rhomboids
Secondary: Hamstrings

Step 1: Lie on your front, with your legs extended straight behind you. Place your hands down by your sides. Keep your eyes fixed on the floor and your neck and head in a neutral position. Engage your abdominals.

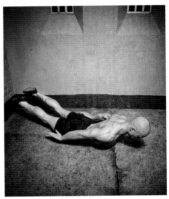

Step 2: Slowly raise your head and chest off the floor, at the same time raise your legs off the floor.

Step 3: Continue the movement, slowly lowering your chest and legs back down to the start position.

Tip: Do not over extend when raising your upper body off the floor.

FULL DORSAL RAISE WITH FINGERS ON TEMPLES

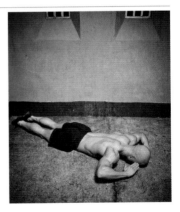

Target Muscle Groups
Primary: Erector Spinae, Gluteus, Rhomboids
Secondary: Hamstrings, Deltoids

Step 1: Lie on your front, with your legs extended straight behind you. Place your fingers on your temples, elbows out wide. Keep your eyes fixed on the floor and your neck and head in a neutral position. Engage your abdominals.

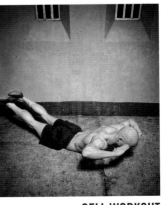

Step 2: Slowly raise your head and chest off the floor, at the same time raise your legs off the floor.

Step 3: Continue the movement, slowly lowering your chest and legs back down to the start position.

SUPERMAN

Target Muscle Groups

Primary: Erector Spinae, Gluteals, Rhomboids

Secondary: Hamstrings, Deltoids, Trapezius

Step 1: Lie on your front, with your legs extended straight behind you and your arms extended straight out in front. Keep your eyes fixed on the floor and your neck and head in a neutral position. Engage your abdominals.

Step 2: Slowly raise your head and chest off the floor, at the same time raise your legs. Maintain contact with your hips on the floor.

Step 3: Continue the movement, slowly lowering your chest and legs back down to the start position.

Tip: For a variation, this exercise can also be performed by placing your arms and legs in a star shape before raising your head and chest off the floor.

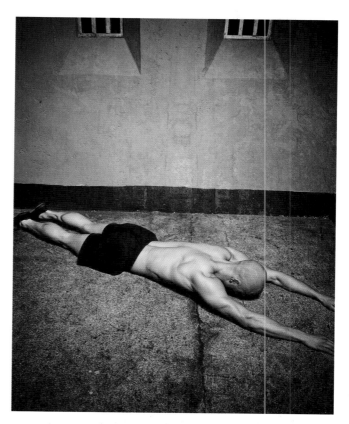

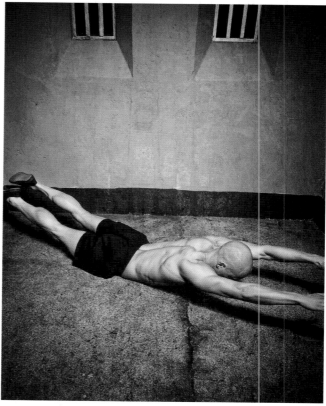

SWIMMER

Target Muscle Groups

Primary: Erector Spinae, Gluteals, Rhomboids

Secondary: Hamstrings, Deltoids, Trapezius

Step 1: Lie on your front, with your legs extended behind you and feet together. Extend your arms out in front. Keep your eyes fixed on the floor and your neck and head in a neutral position. Engage your abdominals.

Step 2: Raise one arm and the opposite leg off the floor, at the same time raising your head and chest, maintaining contact with your hips on the floor.

Step 3: Continue the movement, alternating the opposite arm and leg.

Tip: To make the exercise easier, try legs only – keep your hands by your temples, with palms flat on the floor.

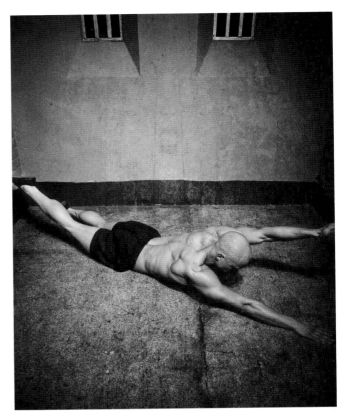

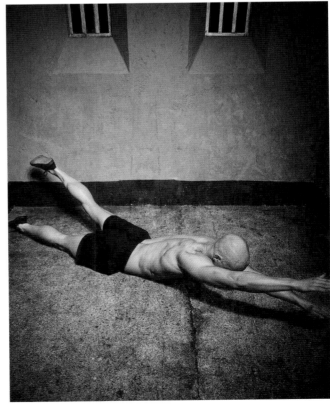

CELL WORKOUT

AIRPLANE

Target Muscle Groups

Primary: Erector Spinae, Gluteals, Rhomboids

Secondary: Hamstrings, Deltoids, Trapezius

Step 1: Lie on your front, with your legs extended straight behind you and your arms extended out to the sides, level with your shoulders. Keep your eyes fixed on the floor and your neck and head in a neutral position. Engage your abdominals.

Step 2: Slowly raise your head, chest and arms off the floor, at the same time raise your legs. Maintain contact with your hips on the floor.

Step 3: Continue the movement, slowly lowering your chest and legs back down to the start position.

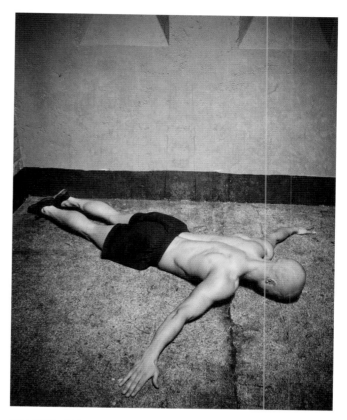

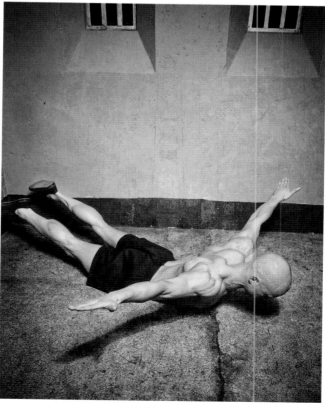

SCAPULAR RETRACTION

Target Muscle Groups
Primary: Rhomboids, Trapezius
Secondary:

Step 1: Stand with your feet hip-width apart, hands on your hips and back relaxed.

Step 2: Open up your chest and pull your shoulder blades back, squeezing your shoulder blades together.

Step 3: Continue the movement, holding the tension for the desired length of time. Release the tension slowly.

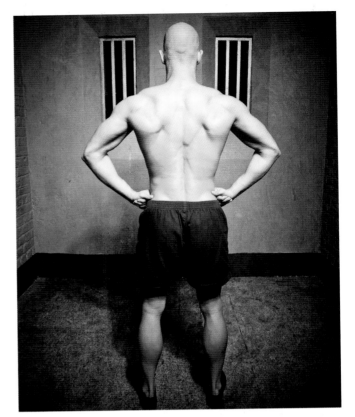

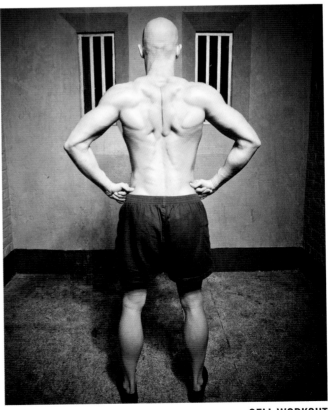

BACK

SCAPULAR RETRACTION WITH BENT ARMS

Target Muscle Groups
Primary: Rhomboids, Trapezius
Secondary: Deltoids

Step 1: Stand with your feet hip-width apart, lift your arms and bend your elbows at a 90-degree angle, up in line with your shoulders and back relaxed.

Step 2: Open up your chest and pull your shoulder blades back, squeezing your shoulder blades together.

Step 3: Continue the movement, holding the tension for the desired length of time. Release the tension slowly.

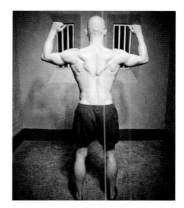

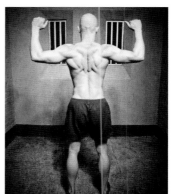

SCAPULAR RETRACTION WITH STRAIGHT ARMS

Target Muscle Groups
Primary: Rhomboids, Trapezius
Secondary: Deltoids

Step 1: Stand with your feet hip-width apart, extend your arms straight out in front of you at shoulder-height and back relaxed.

Step 2: Open up your chest and extending your arms out to the sides, inline with your shoulders. Squeeze your shoulder blades together.

Step 3: Continue the movement, holding the tension for the desired length of time. Release the tension slowly.

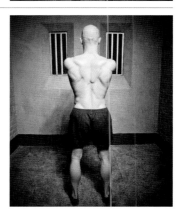

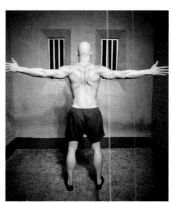

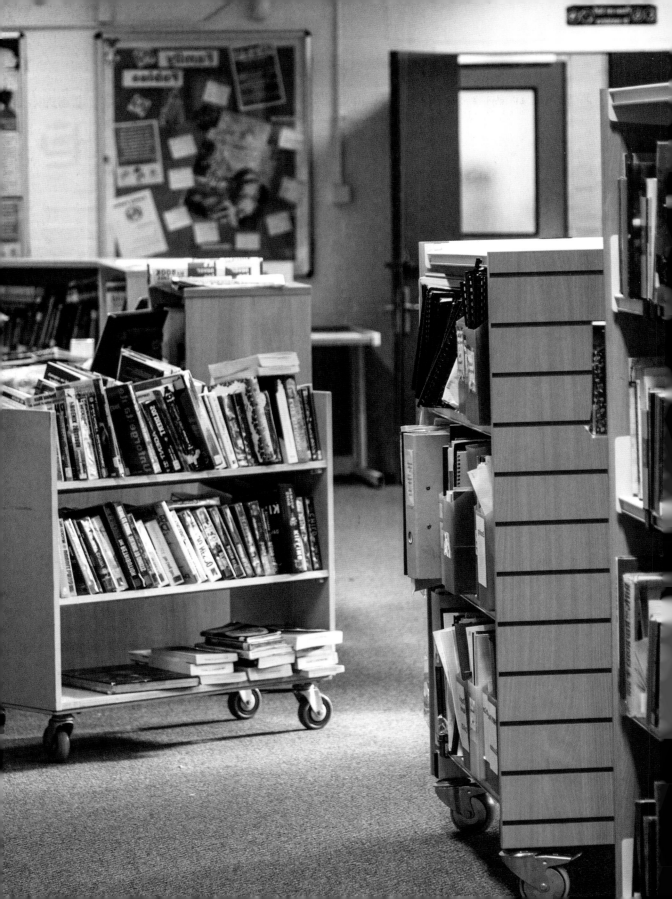

ABDOMINALS & OBLIQUES

The abdomen is situated between the lower part of the rib cage and the upper part of the pelvis. The abdominal and oblique muscles are within this area. These are extremely important as they protect your internal organs, support your core and also allow you to cough and sneeze.

MUSCLE GROUPS

Abdominals

Rectus Abdominis
This is a long flat muscle, which lies at the front of the abdomen. These are more commonly known as 'the abs' and give the '6-pack' appearance.

Basic function: *to flex the spine, compress the contents of the abdomen, and tense the abdominal wall for support and protection.*

Transverse Abdominis
This is a wide horizontal muscle, which originates from the flanks of the body and sits on top of the rectus abdominis and blends into the midline of the rectus abdominis.

Basic function: *to compress abdominal contents.*

Obliques
The obliques are located on the side of the abdomen starting from the lower ribs and down to the top of the pelvis. They are split into two groups; external and internal.

External Obliques
This is the most superficial muscle group on the flank, which when defined, gives the appearance of finger like projections on the lower ribs because the muscle fibres point inwards and downwards towards the pelvis.

Basic function: *flexes the trunk from side to side, to compress abdominal contents.*

Internal Obliques
These lie deeper than the external obliques and are smaller and thinner. They are located slightly lower on the flank.

Basic function: *the same as external obliques.*

CRUNCH

Target Muscle Groups
Primary: Abdominals
Secondary:

Step 1: Lie on your back with knees bent and feet flat on the floor, hip-width apart. Touch your temples with your fingertips, keeping your elbows out wide.

Step 2: Engage your abdominals. Maintain a neutral position with your head and back, and a space between your chin and chest. Look up at the ceiling as you slowly raise your shoulders off the floor, towards your thighs.

Step 3: Continue the movement, slowly lowering back down to the start position.

Tips: When performing exercises where you are lying with your back flat on the floor, avoid arching your lower back and lifting it off the floor.

Keep a space between your chin and chest as you lift your shoulders off the floor.

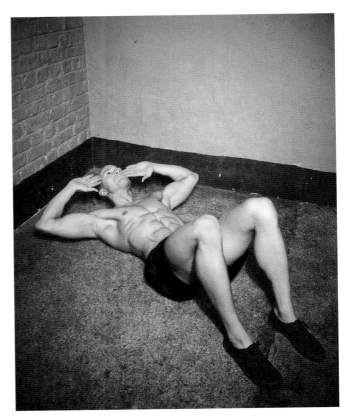

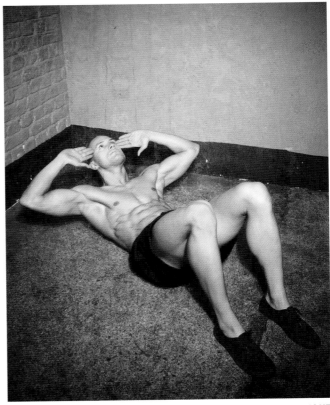

CRUNCH WITH RAISED BENT KNEES

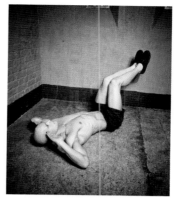

Target Muscle Groups
Primary: Abdominals
Secondary: Quadriceps

Step 1: Lie on your back, with your knees bent to a 90- degree angle, so that your knees are directly over your hips and your feet are raised off the ground. Touch your temples with your fingertips, keeping your elbows out wide.

Step 2: Engage your abdominals. Maintain a neutral position with your head and back, and a space between your chin and chest. Look up at the ceiling as you slowly raise your shoulders off the floor, towards your thighs.

Step 3: Continue the movement, slowly lowering back down to the start position.

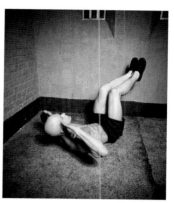

Tip: You can also perform this exercise with your hands behind your head to support your neck, elbows wide.

CRUNCH WITH VERTICAL STRAIGHT LEGS

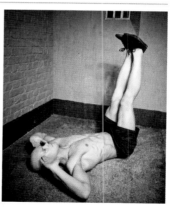

Target Muscle Groups
Primary: Abdominals
Secondary: Quadriceps, Hamstrings

Step 1: Lie on your back, with your legs extended straight up towards the ceiling and feet flexed. Touch your temples with your fingertips, keeping your elbows out wide.

Step 2: Engage your abdominals. Maintain a neutral position with your head and back, and a space between your chin and chest. Look up at the ceiling as you slowly raise your shoulders off the floor, towards your thighs.

Step 3: Continue the movement, slowly lowering back down to the start position.

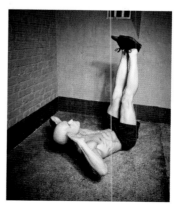

VERTICAL TOE REACH

Target Muscle Groups
Primary: Abdominals
Secondary: Quadriceps, Hamstrings

Step 1: Lie on your back with your legs extended straight up towards the ceiling and feet flexed. Extend your arms straight, in line with your shoulders.

Step 2: Engage your abdominals. Maintain a neutral position with your head and back, and a space between your chin and chest. Look up at the ceiling as you slowly raise your shoulders off the floor and reach your hands towards your feet.

Step 3: Continue the movement, slowly lowering back down to the start position.

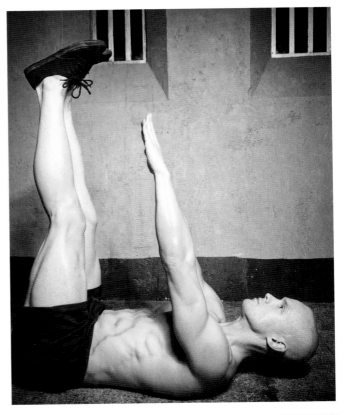

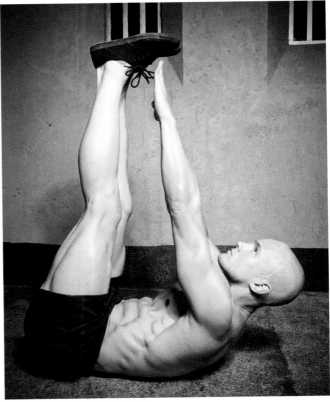

OPPOSITE VERTICAL TOE REACH

Target Muscle Groups
Primary: Abdominals, Obliques

Secondary: Quadriceps, Hamstrings

Step 1: Lie on your back with your legs extended straight up towards the ceiling and feet flexed. Extend your arms straight up, inline with your shoulders.

Step 2: Engage your abdominals. Maintain a neutral position with your head and back, and a space between your chin and chest. Look up at the ceiling as you slowly raise your shoulders off the floor and reach one hand towards the opposite foot.

Step 3: Continue the movement, slowly lowering back down to the start position. Repeat, reaching the other hand across to the opposite foot.

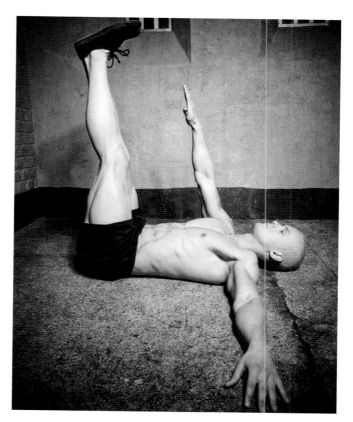

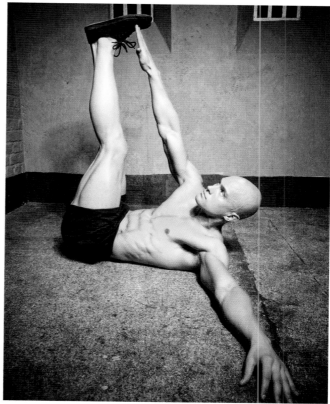

SINGLE LEG RAISE WITH RESTING BENT LEG

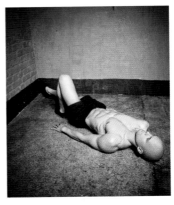

Target Muscle Groups
Primary: Abdominals
Secondary: Quadriceps

Step 1: Lie on your back with one leg bent and foot flat on the floor. Extend the other leg straight out on the floor. Place your arms down by your sides.

Step 2: Engage your abdominals and keeping your lower back in contact with the floor, lift the straight leg off the floor, keeping the bent leg still.

Step 3: Continue the movement, slowly lowering your leg back down without touching the floor. Repeat,then alternate using the opposite leg.

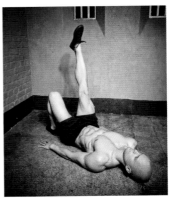

SINGLE LEG RAISE WITH VERTICAL STRAIGHT LEG

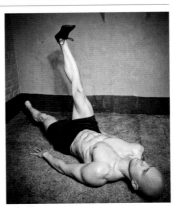

Target Muscle Groups
Primary: Abdominals
Secondary: Quadriceps

Step 1: Lie on your back, with one leg extended straight up towards the ceiling and the other leg straight on the floor. Place your arms by your sides.

Step 2: Engage your abdominals and and keeping your lower back in contact with the floor, slowly raise the lower leg straight up until it is up inline with the raised leg.

Step 3: Continue the movement, slowly lowering the leg without touching the floor. Repeat, raising the opposite leg.

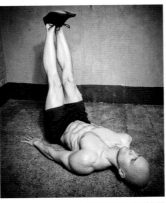

DOUBLE LEG RAISE

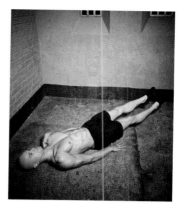

Target Muscle Groups
Primary: Abdominals
Secondary: Quadriceps

Step 1: Lie on your back, with your legs extended straight out on the floor. Place your arms straight by your sides.

Step 2: Engage your abdominals and keeping your lower back in contact with the floor, slowly raise both legs off the floor, towards the ceiling.

Step 3: Continue the movement, slowly lowering your legs down without touching the floor.

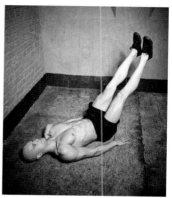

Tip: Only lift and lower your legs as far as your abdominals have sufficient strength for, making sure your lower back maintains contact with the floor.

DOUBLE LEG RAISE WITH LOW RANGE

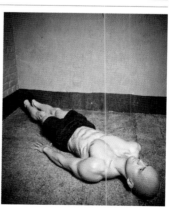

Target Muscle Groups
Primary: Abdominals
Secondary: Quadriceps

Step 1: Lie on your back, with your legs extended straight out on the floor. Place your arms straight by your sides.

Step 2: Engage your abdominals and keeping your lower back in contact with the floor, slowly raise both legs a few inches off the floor.

Step 3: Continue the movement, slowly lowering your legs down without touching the floor.

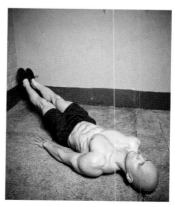

LYING KNEE TUCK WITH SINGLE LEG

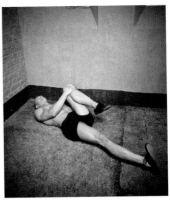

Target Muscle Groups
Primary: Abdominals
Secondary: Quadriceps

Step 1: Lie flat on the floor, holding one knee tucked in towards the chest. Extend the other leg out straight, raised slightly off the floor, with your foot flexed.

Step 2: Engage your abdominals. Look up towards the ceiling, pushing through the heel of your bent leg as you extend it out straight, while at the same time bringing the straight leg in towards your chest.

Step 3: Continue the movement, alternating your leg positions, without touching the straight leg down on the floor.

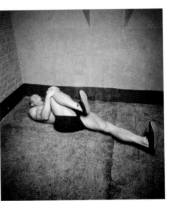

SHOULDERS RAISED LYING KNEE TUCK WITH SINGLE LEG

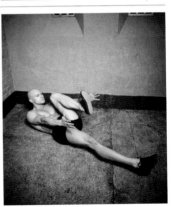

Target Muscle Groups
Primary: Abdominals
Secondary: Quadriceps

Step 1: Lie flat on the floor, with one knee bent, tucked in towards your chest. Extend the other leg out straight with your foot flexed, raised slightly off the floor. Extend your arms out straight in front.

Step 2: Engage your abdominals. Raise your head and shoulders towards your knee, pushing through the heel of your bent leg as you extend it out straight, while at the same time bringing the straight leg in towards your chest.

Step 3: Continue the movement, alternating your leg positions, without touching your straight leg down on the floor.

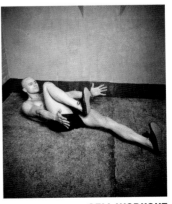

SEATED KNEE TUCK WITH SINGLE LEG

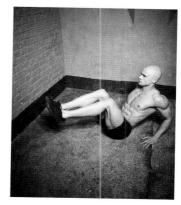

Target Muscle Groups
Primary: Abdominals
Secondary: Quadriceps

Step 1: Sit, leaning back and resting on your hands placed behind you, with your elbows bent. Bend both legs up in front of your chest.

Step 2: Engage your abdominals, keep your upper body still and press through the heel of one leg, pushing it out straight in front of you.

Step 3: Continue the movement, bringing the extended leg back in while pushing the other leg out straight.

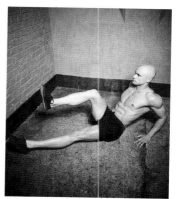

SEATED KNEE TUCK WITH DOUBLE LEG

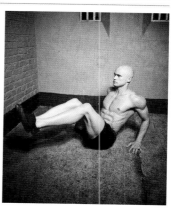

Target Muscle Groups
Primary: Abdominals
Secondary: Quadriceps

Step 1: Sit, leaning back and resting on your hands placed behind you with your elbows bent. Bend both legs up in front of your chest, feet flexed.

Step 2: Engage your abdominals and continue to look straight ahead. Pressing through your heels, extend both legs straight out, without touching the floor.

Step 3: Continue the movement, bringing both knees in towards your chest.

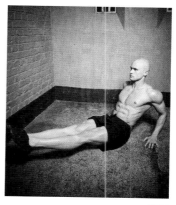

FLUTTER KICK

Target Muscle Groups
Primary: Abdominals
Secondary: Quadriceps

Step 1: Lie on your back, with one leg extended straight up towards the ceiling and the other leg straight on the floor. Place your arms by your sides.

Step 2: Engage your abdominals and maintain a neutral position with your lower back in contact with the floor. Lift and lower the legs, alternating the positions simultaneously.

Step 3: Continue the movement, without touching your legs on the floor.

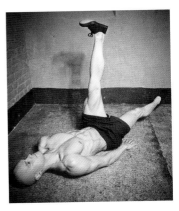

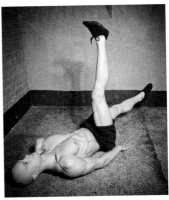

REVERSE CRUNCH

Target Muscle Groups
Primary: Abdominals
Secondary: Quadriceps

Step 1: Lie on your back, with your knees bent to a 90-degree angle, so that your knees are directly over your hips. Place your arms straight by your sides with palms flat on the floor.

Step 2: Engage your abdominals. Pushing down through your palms and keeping your knees bent, curl your hips and back off the floor. Lift your knees until they are inline above your head and you are resting on your shoulders.

Step 3: Continue the movement, slowly curling your spine down to lower your body and legs back down to the start position.

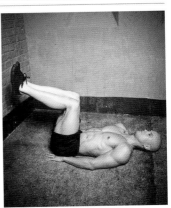

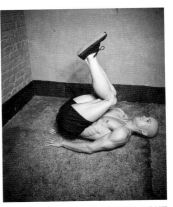

HIP THRUST

Target Muscle Groups
Primary: Abdominals
Secondary: Quadriceps

Step 1: Lie on the floor with legs extended straight up, in line with your hips and feet flexed. Place your arms straight by your sides with palms flat on the floor.

Step 2: Engage your abdominals. Pushing down through your palms, slowly lift your hips off the floor towards the ceiling.

Step 3: Continue the movement, slowly lowering your hips to return to the start position.

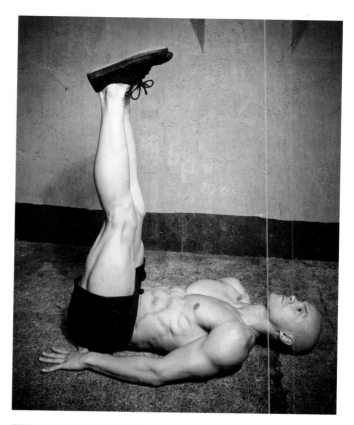

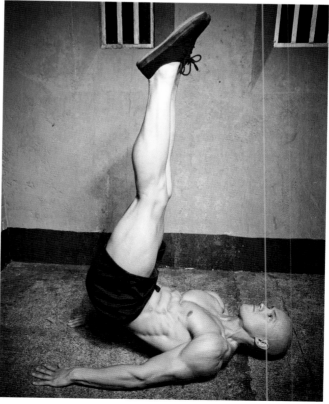

HIGH SCISSORS

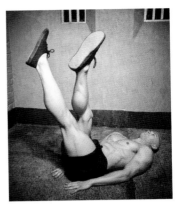

Target Muscle Groups
Primary: Abdominals
Secondary: Quadriceps, Adductors

Step 1: Lie on your back, with your legs extended straight up towards the ceiling, inline with your hips. Place your arms by your sides, palms down.

Step 2: Engage your abdominals and maintain a neutral position, with your lower back in contact with the floor. Look up to the ceiling and, keeping your legs straight and up high, cross them over each other.

Step 3: Continue the movement, alternating the positions to perform a scissor action simultaneously.

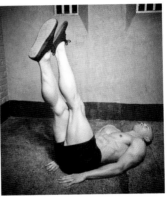

LOW SCISSORS

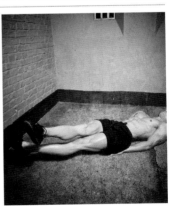

Target Muscle Groups
Primary: Abdominals
Secondary: Quadriceps, Adductors

Step 1: Lie on your back, with your legs extended straight out in front with heels off the floor. Place your arms by your sides, palms down.

Step 2: Engage your abdominals and maintain a neutral position, with your lower back in contact with the floor. Look up to the ceiling and, keeping your legs straight, cross them over each other, in and out.

Step 3: Continue the movement, alternating the positions to perform a scissor action simultaneously.

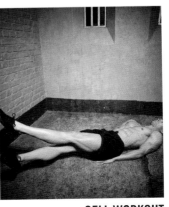

STANDING CRUNCH PULL

Target Muscle Groups
Primary: Abdominals
Secondary: Quadriceps

Step 1: Stand with your feet hip-width apart and your arms extended straight out in front, at shoulder-height.

Step 2: Raise one knee towards your chest and at the same time bend forwards towards the knee and pull your elbows back in towards your sides.

Step 3: Continue the movement, returning your leg and arms back to the upright start position. Repeat, using the other leg.

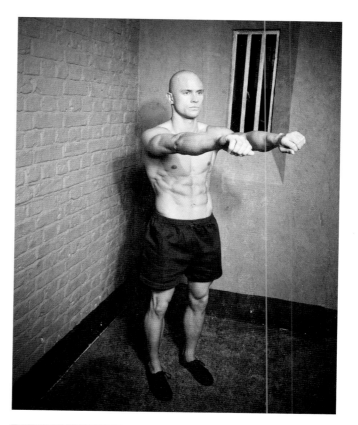

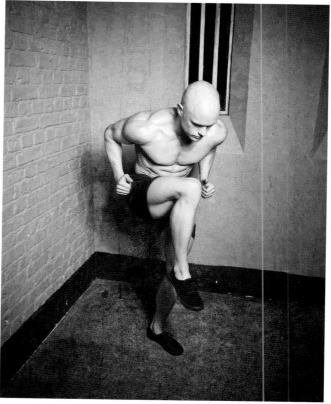

STANDING OBLIQUE TWIST

Target Muscle Groups

Primary: Obliques, Abdominals
Secondary: Quadriceps

Step 1: Stand with your feet hip-width apart and your fingers by your temples.

Step 2: Bend one leg and bring your knee up towards your chest. At the same time, twist at the waist and rotate round to bring the opposite elbow towards the raised knee.

Step 3: Continue the movement, rotating back to return to the upright start position. Repeat, rotating to the other side.

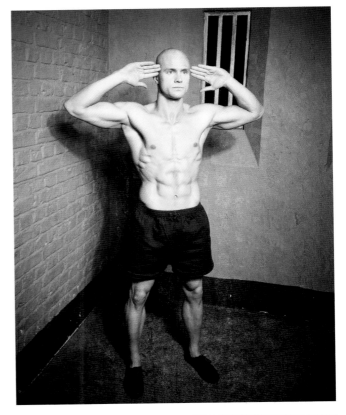

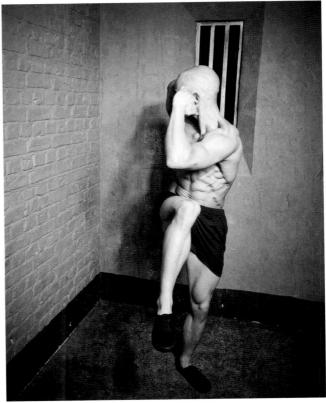

WAIST PINCH

Target Muscle Groups
Primary: Obliques
Secondary: Quadriceps

Step 1: Stand with your feet shoulder-width apart. Place one hand on your hip and one hand by your temple.

Step 2: Bend at the waist and lower your upper elbow down. At the same time lift the knee out to the side to touch your elbow.

Step 3: Continue the movement, straightening your upper body and lower your leg down to tap your toe on the floor. Repeat, then alternate on the other side

Tip: Targets your obliques for a more defined waistline.

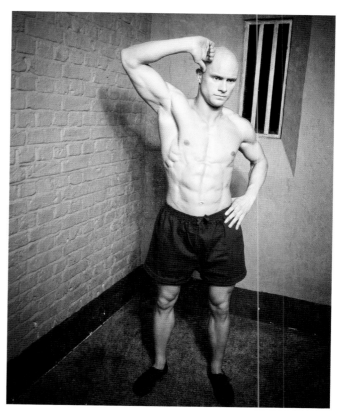

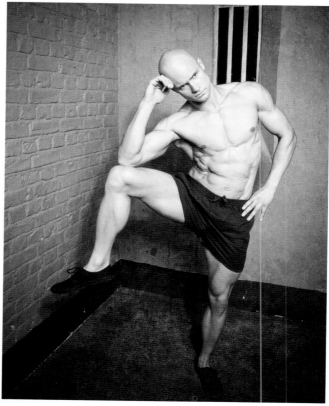

OBLIQUE CRUNCH

Target Muscle Groups
Primary: Obliques, Abdominals
Secondary:

Step 1: Lie on your back, with your knees bent, feet flat on the floor, hip-width apart. Place your fingers on your temples, with your elbows bent and out wide. Maintain a neutral position with your head and back, and a space between your chin and chest.

Step 2: Engage your abdominals and, leading with your chin and chest, raise your shoulders off the floor. Rotate your upper body to reach across your body, taking one elbow towards the opposite knee.

Step 3: Continue the movement, lowering back down to start position. Repeat, reaching the opposite elbow across towards the opposite knee.

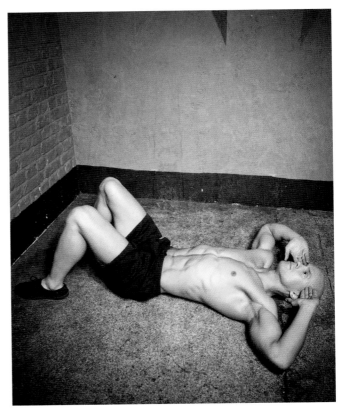

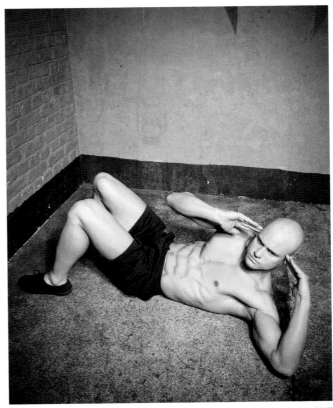

ABDOMINALS & OBLIQUES

132

OBLIQUE CRUNCH WITH RAISED BENT KNEES

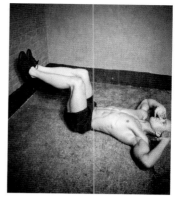

Target Muscle Groups
Primary: Obliques, Abdominals
Secondary: Quadriceps

Step 1: Lie on your back. Raise your legs and bend your knees to a 90-degree angle, so that your knees are directly in line with your hips. Place your fingers on your temples, with your elbows bent and out wide.

Step 2: Engage your abdominals and, leading with your chin and chest, raise your shoulders off the floor. Rotate your upper body to reach across your body, taking one elbow towards the opposite knee.

Step 3: Continue the movement, lowering back down to start position. Repeat, reaching the opposite elbow across towards the opposite knee.

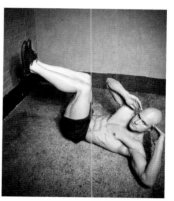

OBLIQUE CRUNCH WITH VERTICAL STRAIGHT LEGS

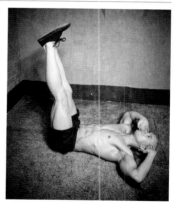

Target Muscle Groups
Primary: Obliques, Abdominals
Secondary: Quadriceps, Hamstrings

Step 1: Lie on your back, with your legs extended straight up in line with your hips. Place your fingers on your temples, with your elbows bent and out wide.

Step 2: Engage your abdominals and, leading with your chin and chest, raise your shoulders off the floor. Rotate your upper body to reach across your body, taking one elbow towards the opposite knee.

Step 3: Continue the movement, lowering back down to the start position. Repeat, reaching the other elbow across towards the opposite knee.

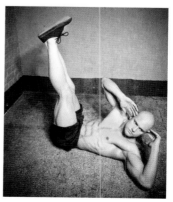

OBLIQUE CRUNCH WITH RESTING BENT LEG

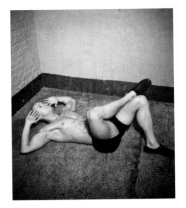

Target Muscle Groups
Primary: Obliques, Abdominals
Secondary: Quadriceps

Step 1: Lie on your back, with one leg bent and foot flat on the floor. Place the other foot across your bent knee. Place your fingers on your temples, with elbows out wide. Maintain a neutral position with your head and back, and a space between your chin and chest.

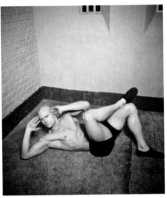

Step 2: Engage your abdominals. Raise your shoulders off the floor and reach across your body to reach the opposite elbow towards the knee of the raised leg.

Step 3: Continue the movement, lowering back down to the start position. Repeat, alternating on the other side.

SIDE LYING OBLIQUE CRUNCH

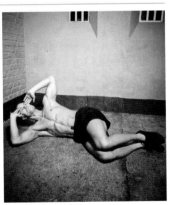

Target Muscle Groups
Primary: Obliques, Abdominals
Secondary:

Step 1: Lie on your side, with your knees bent to 45-degrees and feet together. Place your hands by your temples, elbows wide.

Step 2: Maintaining your side position, lift your upper body and reach your upper elbow down towards your hips.

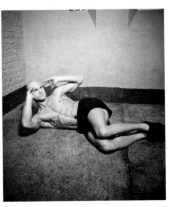

Step 3: Continue the movement, slowly lowering back down to the start position. Repeat, then lie on the other side.

Tip: The main emphasis is on your obliques.

HEEL TAP

Target Muscle Groups
Primary: Obliques, Abdominals
Secondary:

Step 1: Lie on your back, with your knees bent, feet flat on the floor, hip-width apart. Place your arms by your sides. Maintain a neutral position with your head and back, and a space between your chin and chest.

Step 2: Engage your abdominals. Look up at the ceiling as you raise your shoulders off the floor and reach one hand down and tap the heel of the foot on the same side.

Step 3: Continue the movement, alternating sides to reach down and tap the other heel.

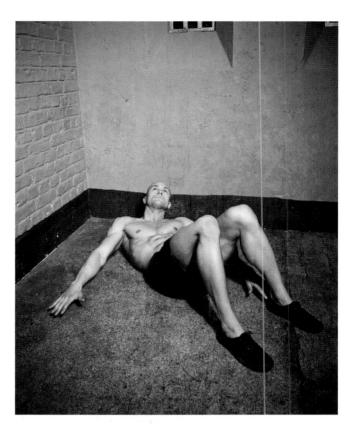

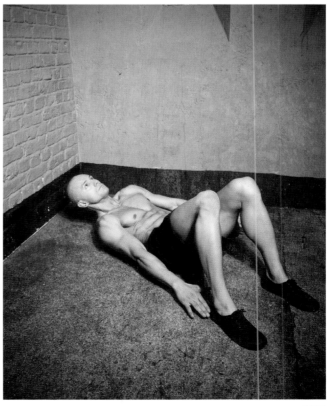

RUSSIAN TWIST WITH BENT ARMS

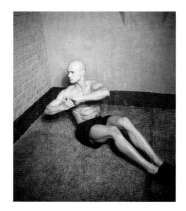

Target Muscle Groups
Primary: Obliques, Abdominals
Secondary: Erector Spinae

Step 1: Sit on the floor with your legs slightly bent in front and feet together. Lean back slightly and clasp your hands in front your chest, elbows out wide.

Step 2: Engage your abdominals. Looking straight ahead, slowly rotate your upper body and arms round to one side.

Step 3: Continue the movement, twisting round to the other side.

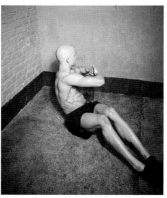

Tips: Leaning your upper body back slightly will help keep you balanced as you rotate during this exercise. Use a slow controlled movement at all times to avoid injury to the back.

You can also perform this exercise with legs raised.

RUSSIAN TWIST WITH STRAIGHT ARMS

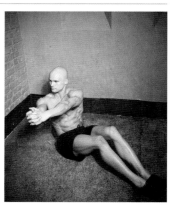

Target Muscle Groups
Primary: Obliques, Abdominals
Secondary: Erector Spinae

Step 1: Sit on the floor with your legs slightly bent in front and feet together. Lean back slightly and extend your arms straight out in front of your chest, with your hands clasped.

Step 2: Engage your abdominals. Looking straight ahead, slowly rotate your upper body and arms round to one side.

Step 3: Continue the movement, twisting round to the other side.

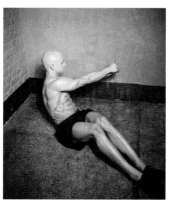

Tips: Leaning your upper body back slightly will help keep you balanced as you rotate during this exercise. Use a slow controlled movement at all times to avoid injury to the back.

ABDOMINALS & OBLIQUES

BICYCLE CRUNCH

Target Muscle Groups
Primary: Obliques, Abdominals
Secondary: Quadriceps

Step 1: Lie on your back, with your knees bent to a 90-degree angle directly in line with your hips. Place your hands by your temples and elbows out wide. Maintain a neutral position with your head and back, and a space between your chin and chest.

Step 2: Engage your abdominals. As you slowly lift your shoulders off the floor, rotate your upper body to reach across your body, taking one elbow towards the opposite knee. At the same time straighten out the opposite leg.

Step 3: Continue the movement, alternating sides and switching the leg positions in a cycling action.

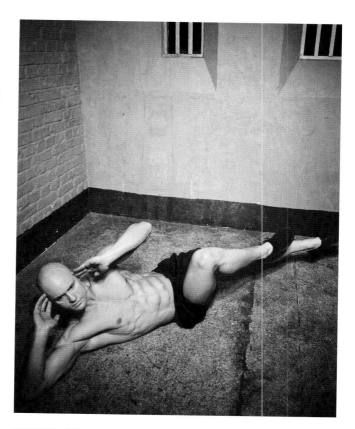

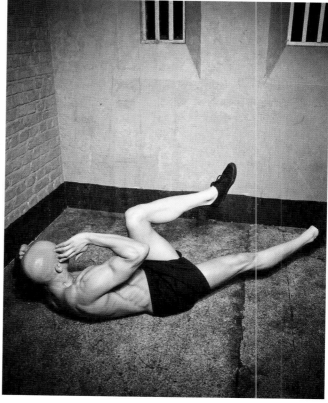

PLANK

Target Muscle Groups
Primary: Abdominals, Erector Spinae
Secondary: Deltoids, Triceps

Step 1: Face down on the floor, with your legs extended behind you hip-width apart, with your toes tucked under. Rest on your forearms and elbows, to form a plank.

Step 2: Engage your abdominals. Maintain proper alignment with your body, forming a straight line from your head to heels.

Step 3: Continue the movement, holding the position for the desired length of time, keeping your body parallel to the ground. Release the tension slowly.

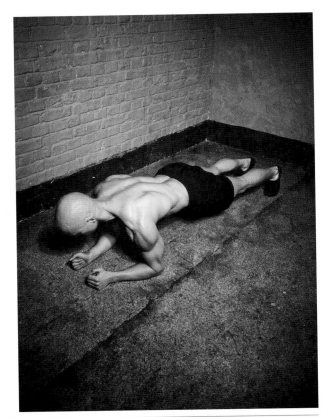

FULL PLANK

Target Muscle Groups
Primary: Abdominals, Erector Spinae
Secondary: Deltoids, Triceps

Step 1: Assume the plank position. Place your hands directly under your shoulders, with your arms straight to form a full plank.

Step 2: Engage your abdominals. Maintain proper alignment with your body, forming a straight line from your head to heels.

Step 3: Continue the movement, holding the position for the desired length of time. Release the tension slowly.

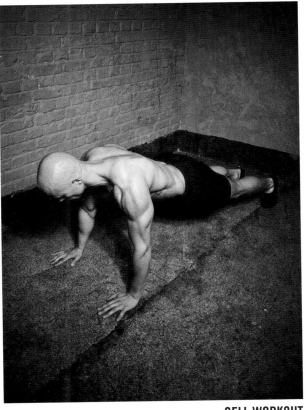

FULL PLANK WITH SINGLE KNEE TUCK

Target Muscle Groups
Primary: Abdominals, Erector Spinae
Secondary: Deltoids, Triceps, Quadriceps

Step 1: Face down on the floor, with your legs extended behind you hip-width apart, with your toes tucked under. Place your hands directly under your shoulders, arms straight, to form a full plank.

Step 2: Maintain proper alignment with your body, forming a straight line from your head to heels. Engage your abdominals as you bring one knee in towards your chest.

Step 3: Continue the movement, returning the leg back to the start position and alternate using the other knee.

Tips: When performing any plank exercise, maintain a straight line without lifting your hips excessively towards the ceiling or letting them sag. Use the strength from your entire core, particularly the abdominals, to hold a steady position.

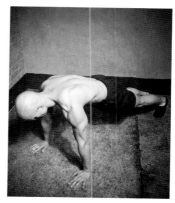
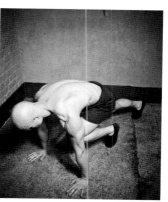

FULL PLANK WITH KNEE TO ELBOW

Target Muscle Groups
Primary: Obliques, Abdominals, Erector Spinae
Secondary: Deltoids, Triceps, Quadriceps

Step 1: Face down on the floor, with your legs extended behind you hip-width apart, with your toes tucked under. Place your hands directly under your shoulders, arms straight, to form a full plank.

Step 2: Maintain proper alignment with your body, forming a straight line from your head to heels. Bend one knee and bring it round towards the elbow on the same side.

Step 3: Continue the movement, returning the leg back to the start position and alternate sides.

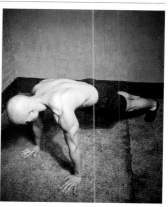
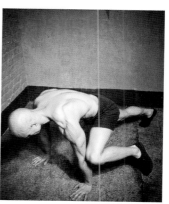

FULL PLANK WITH OPPOSITE KNEE TO ELBOW

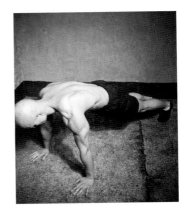

Target Muscle Groups
Primary: Obliques, Abdominals, Erector Spinae
Secondary: Deltoids, Triceps, Quadriceps

Step 1: Face down on the floor, with your legs extended behind you hip-width apart, with your toes tucked under. Place your hands directly under your shoulders, arms straight, to form a full plank.

Step 2: Engage your abdominals, as you bring one knee in towards your chest. When your knee is tucked up under your chest, twist it under your body, to reach towards the opposite elbow, so that your upper body also twists.

Step 3: Continue the movement, returning the leg back to the start position and alternate to twist to the opposite elbow.

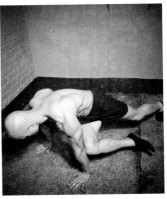

FULL PLANK SWEEP

Target Muscle Groups
Primary: Obliques, Abdominals, Erector Spinae
Secondary: Deltoids, Triceps, Quadriceps

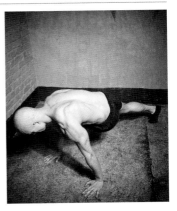

Step 1: Face down on the floor, with your legs extended behind you hip-width apart, with your toes tucked under. Place your hands directly under your shoulders, arms straight, to form a full plank.

Step 2: Engage your abdominals, as you bring one knee in towards your chest. When your knee is tucked up under your chest, twist it under your body, to reach towards the opposite elbow, so that your upper body also twists.

Step 3: Continue the movement, sweeping your knee out across your body to the outside of your other elbow. Return to the start position. Repeat, alternating sides.

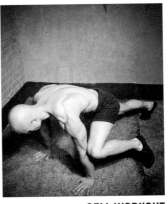

SIDE PLANK

Target Muscle Groups
Primary: Obliques
Secondary: Abdominals, Deltoids

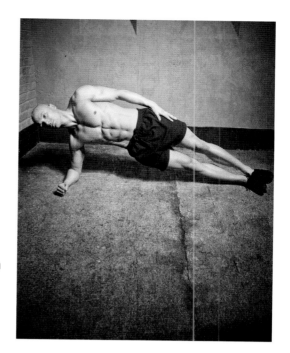

Step 1: Lie on your side, with your legs straight and feet together. Rest on the forearm of your lower arm, with your elbow directly under your shoulder and your other arm by your side.

Step 2: Engage your abdominals and look straight ahead. Maintain a straight line with your head, neck and body. Push down through your forearm and feet, to raise your hips off the floor and your legs are straight.

Step 3: Continue the movement, holding the position for the desired length of time. Release the tension slowly. Repeat, alternating sides.

SIDE PLANK WITH STRAIGHT ARM

Target Muscle Groups
Primary: Obliques
Secondary: Abdominals, Deltoids, Triceps

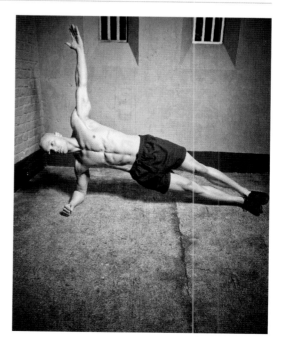

Step 1: Assume a side plank position. Extend your upper arm straight up towards the ceiling, in line with your shoulder.

Step 2: Engage your abdominals and look straight ahead. Maintain a straight line with your head, neck and body as you push down through your forearm and feet, to raise your body up until your legs are straight.

Step 3: Continue the movement, holding the position for the desired length of time. Release the tension slowly. Repeat, alternating sides.

SIDE PLANK WITH TORSO ROTATION

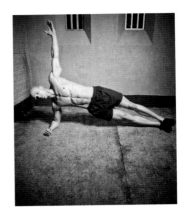

Target Muscle Groups
Primary: Obliques
Secondary: Abdominals, Erector Spinae, Deltoids

Step 1: Lie on your side with your legs straight and feet together. Rest on the forearm of your lower arm on the floor, with your elbow directly under your shoulder and extend your other arm straight up towards the ceiling, in line with your shoulder.

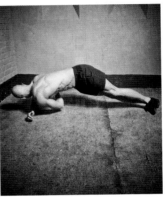

Step 2: Engage your abdominals and look straight ahead. Maintain a straight line with your head, neck and body as you push down through your forearm and feet, to raise your body up until your legs are straight.

Step 3: Rotate your body as you bring the extended arm down and reach underneath your upper body.

Step 4: Continue the movement, rotating back to the start position. Repeat, then alternate sides.

SIDE PLANK WITH LEG LIFT

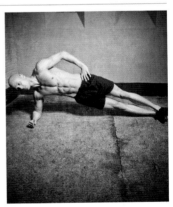

Target Muscle Groups
Primary: Obliques
Secondary: Abdominals, Deltoids, Quadriceps

Step 1: Lie on your side with your legs straight and feet together. Rest on the forearm of your lower arm on the floor, with your elbow directly under your shoulder and place your other hand on your hip.

Step 2: Engage your abdominals. Maintain a straight line with your head, neck and body as you push down through your forearm and feet, to raise your body up until your legs are straight.

Step 3: Lift the upper leg up in line with your hips, keeping the rest of your body still.

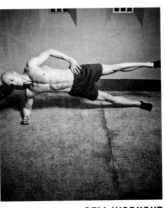

Step 4: Continue the movement, lowering your leg back down to the start position. Repeat, then alternate sides.

SIDE PLANK WITH LEG LIFT AND FRONT KICK

Target Muscle Groups
Primary: Obliques
Secondary: Abdominals, Deltoids, Quadriceps

Step 1: Lie on your side with your legs straight and feet together. Rest on the forearm of your lower arm on the floor, with your elbow directly under your shoulder and place your other hand on your hip.

Step 2: Engage your abdominals and look straight ahead. Maintain a straight line with your head, neck and body as you push down through your forearm and feet, to raise your body up until your legs are straight.

Step 3: Lift the upper leg up in line with your hips, then kick your leg forwards, keeping the rest of your body still.

Step 4: Continue the movement, lowering your leg back down to the start position. Repeat, then alternate sides.

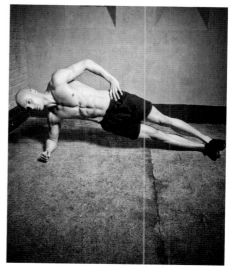

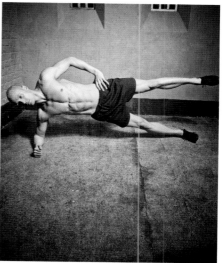

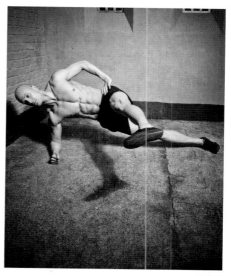

SIDE PLANK WITH OBLIQUE CRUNCH

Target Muscle Groups
Primary: Obliques
Secondary: Abdominals, Deltoids, Quadriceps

Step 1: Lie on your side with your legs straight and feet together. Rest on the forearm of your lower arm on the floor, with your elbow directly under your shoulder and place the hand of your upper arm by your temple.

Step 2: Engage your abdominals. Maintain a straight line with your head, neck and body as you push down through your forearm and feet, to raise your body up until your legs are straight.

Step 3: Bend the knee of your upper leg and bring it up towards your shoulder. At the same time bend your upper elbow down to touch the knee.

Step 4: Continue the movement, rotating back to the start position. Repeat, then alternate sides.

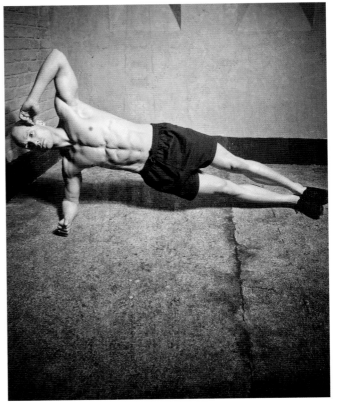

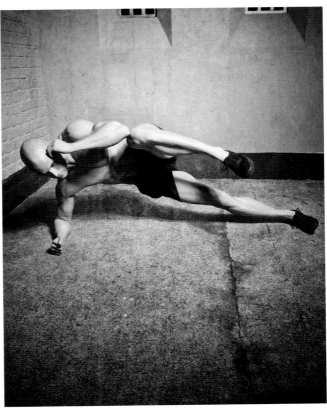

SIDE PLANK WITH OPPOSITE OBLIQUE CRUNCH

Target Muscle Groups
Primary: Obliques
Secondary: Abdominals, Deltoids, Quadriceps

Step 1: Lie on your side with your legs straight and feet together. Rest on the forearm of your lower arm on the floor, with your elbow directly under your shoulder and place the hand of your upper arm by your temple.

Step 2: Engage your abdominals. Maintain a straight line with your head, neck and body as you push down through your forearm and feet, to raise your body up until your legs are straight.

Step 3: Bend the knee of your lower leg and bring it up towards your chest. At the same time bend your upper elbow down to touch the knee.

Step 4: Continue the movement, returning back to the start position. Repeat, then alternate sides.

Tip: For a harder version, straighten your supporting arm.

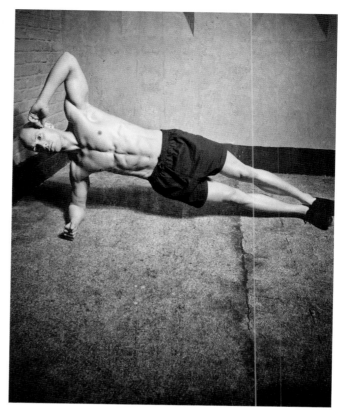

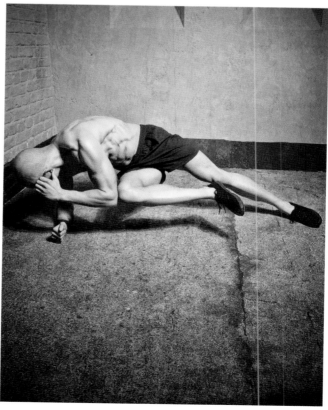

FULL SIDE PLANK

Target Muscle Groups
Primary: Obliques
Secondary: Abdominals, Deltoids, Triceps

Step 1: Lie on your side with your legs straight and feet together. Straighten your lower arm, with your hand directly under your shoulder and rest your other arm by your side.

Step 2: Engage your abdominals. Maintain a straight line with your head, neck and body as you push down through your lower hand and feet, to raise your body up until your legs are straight.

Step 3: Continue the movement, holding the position for the desired length of time. Release the tension slowly. Repeat, then alternate sides.

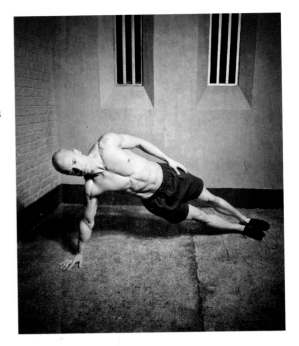

FULL SIDE PLANK WITH STRAIGHT ARM

Target Muscle Groups
Primary: Obliques
Secondary: Abdominals, Deltoids, Triceps

Step 1: Assume a full side plank with straight arm position. Extend the upper arm, in line with your shoulder, straight up towards the ceiling.

Step 2: Maintain a straight line with your head, neck and body as you push down through your arm and feet, to lift your body up until your arms and legs are straight.

Step 3: Continue the movement, holding the position for the desired length of time. Release the tension slowly. Repeat, then alternate sides.

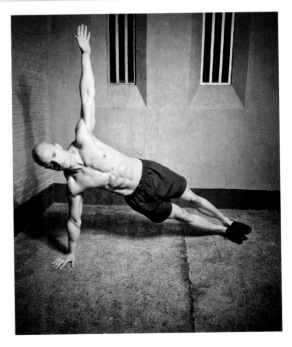

FULL SIDE PLANK WITH LEG LIFT

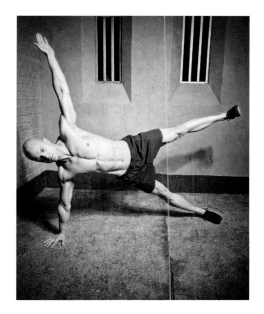

Target Muscle Groups
Primary: Obliques
Secondary: Abdominals, Deltoids, Triceps, Quadriceps

Step 1: Assume a full side plank with straight arm position.

Step 2: Maintain a straight line with your head, neck and body, as you push down through your arm and feet, to lift your body up until your arms and legs are straight.

Step 3: Lift the upper leg up inline with your hips, keeping the rest of your body still.

Step 4: Continue the movement, holding the position for the desired length of time. Release the tension slowly. Repeat, then alternate sides.

FULL SIDE PLANK WITH TORSO ROTATION

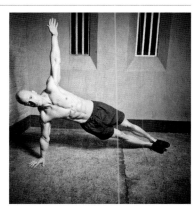

Target Muscle Groups
Primary: Obliques
Secondary: Abdominals, Deltoids, Triceps

Step 1: Assume a full side plank with straight arm position. Extend the upper arm, in line with your shoulder, straight up towards the ceiling.

Step 2: Maintain a straight line with your head, neck and body, as you push down through your arm and feet, to lift your body up until your arms and legs are straight.

Step 3: Rotate your body as you bring the extended arm down and reach underneath your upper body.

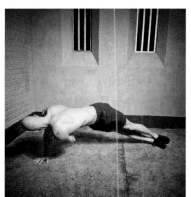

Step 4: Continue the movement, rotating back to the start position. Repeat, then alternate sides.

LEGS

There are two main functions of the lower limb. Firstly, to support the weight of the body with minimal expenditure of energy. Secondly, locomotion in humans. Other functions include engaging in other activities such as kicking a ball or jumping.

The leg is made up of numerous bones and joints. Starting from the top of the leg: at the hip, the thigh bone (femur) inserts into the pelvis in a ball and socket joint. Moving down the leg, at the knee, the femur meets the bones of the lower leg (tibia and fibula) and forms a hinge joint, with the kneecap lying on top of it. Finally, the tibia and fibula meet the bones of the foot at the ankle forming another hinge joint.

MUSCLE GROUPS

There are a number of muscles in the leg:

Quadriceps
The quadriceps are made from four large muscles: rectus femoris, vastus lateralis, vastus medialis, vastus intermedius, more commonly known as the 'quads'. They are located on the front of the thigh. They work together to perform the same function. The vastus muscles orginate from the top of the femur, while the longer rectus femoris originates from the pelvis, however they all attach around the knee joint.

Basic function: *mainly to extend (straighten) the leg at the knee and stabilise the kneecap.*

Hamstrings
There are three long muscles at the back of the thigh, collectively known as the hamstrings. They all originate at the pelvis and attach at the back of the knee. The three muscles are biceps femoris, semitendinosus and semimembranosus. The bicep femoris has two heads: one long and one short.

Basic function: *flexes the leg at the knee joint (bends the knee – brings foot to glutes), and extend the leg at the hip joint (straightens leg backwards). They are also involved in rotation at both of these joints.*

Adductors
While the quadriceps and hamstrings are at the front and back of the thigh respectively, the adductors are located on the inner side of the thigh. There are six muscles that collectively work together to perform a variety of functions.

Basic function: adduct the thigh (move leg inwards, towards the body at the hip joint), and also rotate the thigh inwards and outwards.

Gluteals
The gluteals (glutes) are made up three muscles: gluteus minimus, gluteus medius and gluteus maximus. This is a large group of muscles and form the most superficial group of the buttock. They originate from the back of the pelvis and attach at the upper part of the femur. Again, like most muscles of the leg, they work together to perform the same function.

Basic function: abduct (move leg sideways, away from the body) and extend the leg at the hip joint (straighten leg backwards).

Calves
The calves are located at the back of the lower leg and are involved in foot movements. The two main muscles are the gastrocnemius and the soleus.

Gastrocnemius
The gastrocnemius is one of the largest muscles of the lower leg and has two heads: the medial and lateral head. It originates from the lower part of the femur and attaches to the heel, forming the Achilles tendon.

Basic function: plantarflexion of the foot (points toes downwards).

Soleus
The soleus is a large flat muscle underneath the gastrocnemius. It originates from the bones in the lower leg and joins the Achilles tendon attaching to the heel. Together with the gastrocnemius it plants the foot at the ankle joint.

Basic function: see gastrocnemius.

SQUAT

Target Muscle Groups
Primary: Quadriceps, Gluteals, Hamstrings
Secondary: Adductors

Step 1: Stand with your feet slightly wider than hip-width apart and toes turned out slightly, keeping them aligned with your knees. Extend your arms straight out in front of you, level with your shoulders. Engage your abdominals to brace your spine. Keep your chest lifted and your chin parallel to the floor.

Step 2: Ease your weight back into your heels, bend your knees and hinge at the hips, shifting them back and down. Your hips and knees should bend simultaneously. Do not arch your lower back. Keep your feet flat and your knees in line with, but not beyond, your toes. Lower yourself until your thighs are parallel to the floor, at a 90-degree angle.

Step 3: Continue the movement, pushing through your heels, keeping your body weight evenly distributed between the balls and heels of both feet. Maintain the position of your back, chest and head as you raise your hips.

Tip: Imagine you are about to sit on a chair as you lower down towards the floor.

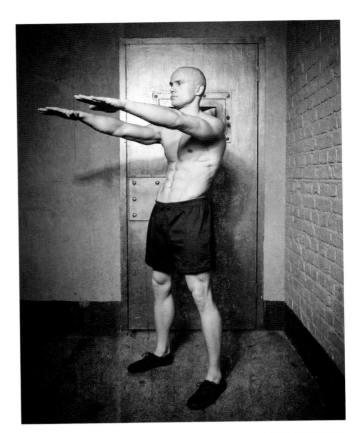

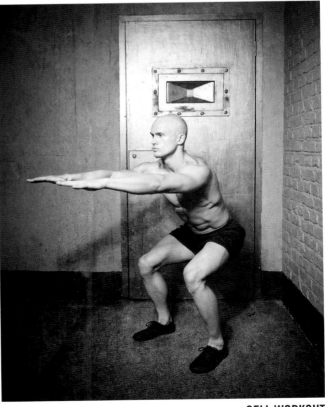

NARROW SQUAT

Target Muscle Groups
Primary: Quadriceps, Gluteals, Hamstrings
Secondary: Adductors

Step 1: From a standing position with feet together, extend your arms straight out in front of you, level with your shoulders.

Step 2: Engage your abdominals, hinge your hips back and lower your upper body down into a squat position, until your thighs are parallel to the floor, squeezing your knees together.

Step 3: Continue the movement, pushing through your heels to slowly raise back up.

Tip: You can perform this exercise with your arms bent at the elbow, in front of your chest and your palms pressed together.

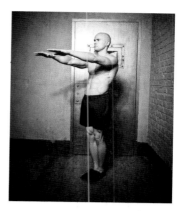

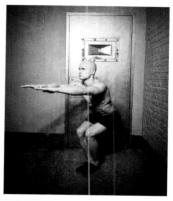

WIDE SQUAT

Target Muscle Groups
Primary: Quadriceps, Gluteals, Hamstrings
Secondary: Adductors

Step 1: Stand with your feet wider than shoulder-width apart. Point your toes slightly outward and keep them aligned with your knees. Extend your arms straight out in front of you, level with your shoulders.

Step 2: Engage your abdominals, hinge your hips back and lower your upper body down into a squat position, until your thighs are parallel to the floor.

Step 3: Continue the movement, pushing through your heels to slowly raising back up.

Tip: Do not position your feet so wide that you lose stability.

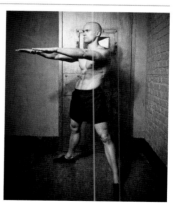

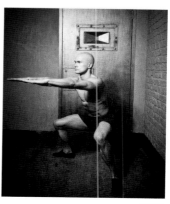

LEGS

PRISONER SQUAT

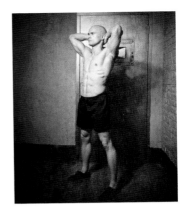

Target Muscle Groups
Primary: Quadriceps, Gluteals, Hamstrings
Secondary: Adductors

Step 1: Stand with your feet wider than shoulder-width apart, point your toes slightly outward and keep them aligned with your knees. Place your hands behind your head. Pull your elbows and shoulders back.

Step 2: Maintain a straight back and engage your abdominals. Hinge your hips back and lower your upper body down, until your thighs are level with your knees, parallel to the floor.

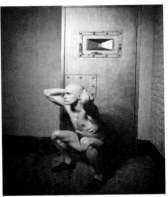

Step 3: Continue the movement, slowly raising back up to the start position, keeping your weight evenly distributed between both feet as you do so and abdominals engaged throughout.

Tip: Taking the squat further down will place more emphasis on your hamstrings and glutes.

SQUAT WITH ROTATION

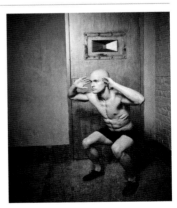

Target Muscle Groups
Primary: Quadriceps, Gluteals, Hamstrings, Obliques
Secondary: Adductors

Step 1: Stand with your feet wider than shoulder-width apart, point your toes slightly outward and keep them aligned with your knees. Pull your elbows and shoulders back and place your fingers on your temples.

Step 2: Hinge your hips back and lower your upper body down into a squat position, until your thighs are parallel to the floor.

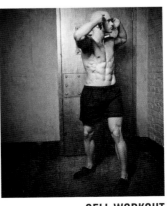

Step 3: Continue the movement slowly raising back up, rotating at the hips to turn your torso to one side. Repeat, rotating to the other side.

SQUAT WITH BENT KNEE LIFT

Target Muscle Groups
Primary: Quadriceps, Gluteals, Hamstrings
Secondary: Adductors, Abdominals

Step 1: Stand with your feet wider than shoulder-width apart, point your toes slightly outward and keep them aligned with your knees. Extend your arms straight out in front of you, level with your shoulders.

Step 2: Hinge your hips back and lower your upper body down into a squat position, until your thighs are parallel to the floor.

Step 3: As you raise back up, lift one knee up in front of your chest and keep your balance.

Step 4: Continue the movement, lowering your foot back down. Repeat, raising the other knee.

Tip: This exercise can also be performed by raising your leg straight out in front or straight out to the side.

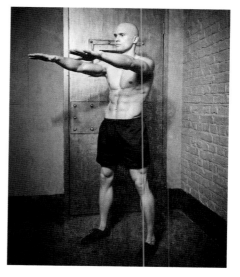
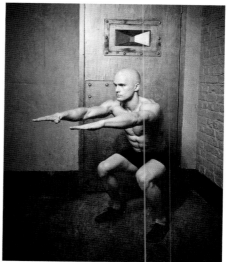
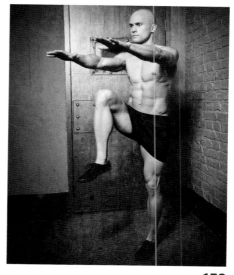

LEGS

WALL SIT

Target Muscle Groups

Primary: Quadriceps, Gluteals

Secondary: Hamstrings, Adductors

Step 1: With your back flat against a wall, your arms by your sides and palms flat against the wall. Lower yourself down until your thighs are parallel to the floor and your knees bent to 90-degrees and in line with your toes, not extended over them.

Step 2: Continue the movement, holding the position for the desired length of time. Slowly raise back up the wall to a standing position.

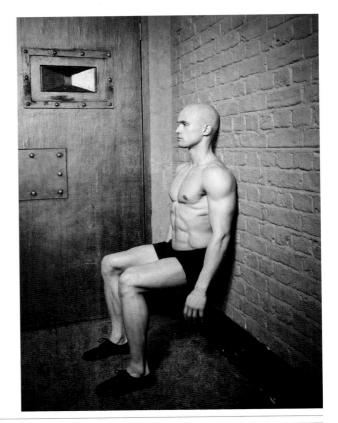

WALL SIT WITH BENT KNEE LIFT

Target Muscle Groups

Primary: Quadriceps, Gluteals

Secondary: Hamstrings, Adductors, Abdominals

Step 1: Assume the wall sit position.

Step 2: Keep your body still and raise one knee up level with your waist.

Step 3: Continue the movement, slowly lowering your foot back down to the floor. Repeat, alternating legs. Slowly raise back up the wall to a standing position.

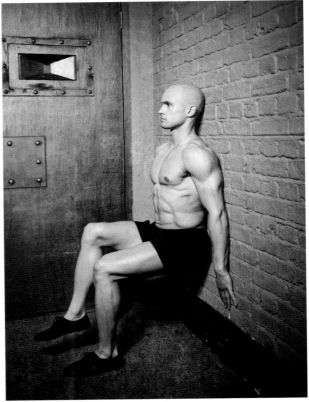

FORWARD LUNGE

Target Muscle Groups
Primary: Quadriceps, Gluteals
Secondary: Hamstrings, Adductors

Step 1: Stand with your feet hip-width apart and your hands on your hips. Pull your shoulder blades down. Engage your abdominals. Maintain a straight back, not leaning forwards or back.

Step 2: Step one foot forward, to form a split-stance.

Step 3: Lower yourself down, bending your front knee, until it is directly over your ankle and your thigh is parallel to the floor, to form a 90-degree angle. At the same time lower your back knee towards the floor.

Step 4: Push up through the front leg and take it back to the start position. Alternate, stepping forwards with the opposite leg.

Tips: Perform a walking version of the lunge by pushing firmly pushing up from the lowered position with your front leg and immediately taking a long step forward with the other leg.

Repeat the movement in a flowing, walking motion. Keep your leading foot fixed as you lower down each time.

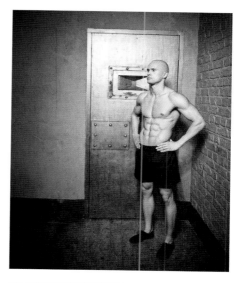
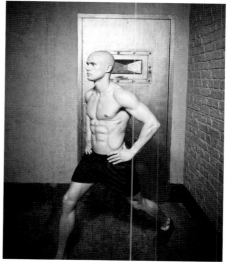
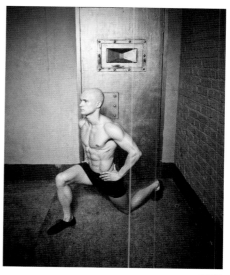

LEGS

REVERSE LUNGE

Target Muscle Groups
Primary: Quadriceps, Gluteals
Secondary: Hamstrings, Adductors

Step 1: Stand with your feet hip-width apart and your hands on your hips. Pull your shoulder blades down towards your hips. Engage your abdominals. Maintain a straight back, not leaning forwards or back.

Step 2: Step one foot back, to form a split-stance.

Step 3: Lower yourself down, bending your front knee, until it is directly over your ankle and your thigh is parallel to the floor, to form a 90-degree angle. At the same time lower your back knee towards the floor.

Step 4: Continue the movement, pushing though your front leg, bringing your back leg forwards to the start position. Repeat, alternating legs.

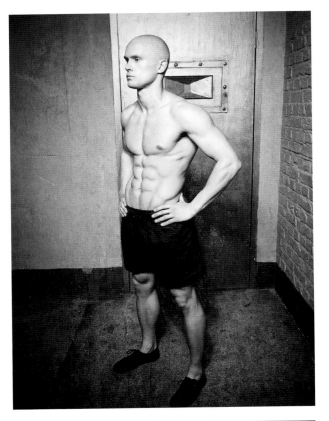

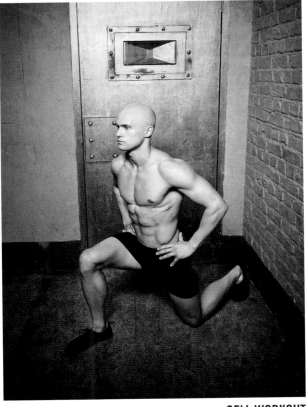

LEGS

DIAGONAL LUNGE

Target Muscle Groups
Primary: Quadriceps, Gluteals
Secondary: Hamstrings, Adductors

Step 1: Stand with your feet hip-width apart and your hands on your hips. Pull your shoulder blades down towards your hips. Engage your abdominals. Keep a straight back, not leaning forwards or back.

Step 2: Step one foot forward, diagonally, to form a split-stance.

Step 3: Lower yourself down, bending your front knee until it is directly over your ankle and your thigh is parallel to the floor, to form a 90-degree angle. At the same time, lower your back knee towards the floor.

Step 4: Continue the movement, push through the front leg and take it backwards to return to the start position. Repeat, stepping forward diagonally with the opposite leg.

Tip: You can also perform this exercise reversing the movement.

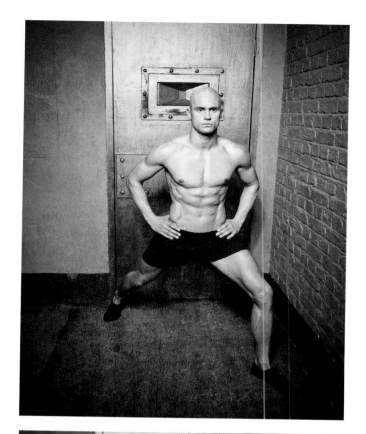

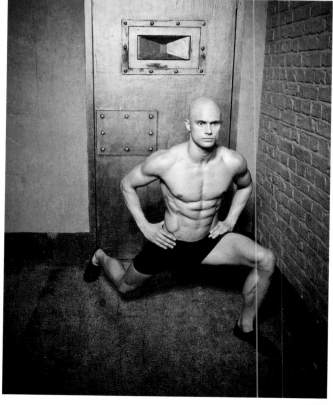

LEGS

LATERAL LUNGE

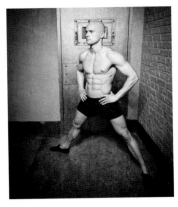

Target Muscle Groups
Primary: Quadriceps, Adductors
Secondary: Gluteals, Hamstrings

Step 1: Stand with your feet in a wide stance and your hands on your hips. Keep your back straight throughout the exercise.

Step 2: Shift your weight to one side and bend your knee. Push your hips back and lower your body, until your bent knee is directly over your ankle, and your weight is pushing through your heels.

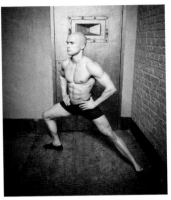

Step 3: Continue the movement, pushing up through the bent leg to return to the start position. Repeat, bending the opposite knee.

LATERAL LUNGE WITH SIDE TOE TOUCH

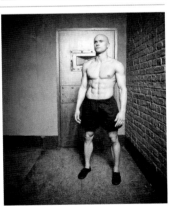

Target Muscle Groups
Primary: Quadriceps, Adductors
Secondary: Gluteals, Hamstrings

Step 1: Stand with your feet hip-width apart and hands down by your sides.

Step 2: Take a wide step out to one side, with your foot pointing outwards. Bend your knee and reach down with both hands to touch the foot of the leg that is bent. Keep the other leg straight throughout.

Step 3: Continue the movement, pushing through your foot back up to the start position. Repeat, taking a wide step out to the opposite side.

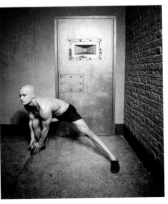

STANDING REAR LEG LIFT

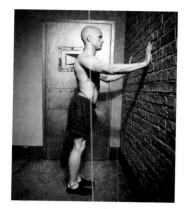

Target Muscle Groups
Primary: Gluteals
Secondary: Hamstrings, Erector Spinae

Step 1: Stand facing a wall with your feet shoulder-width apart. Place your hands flat onto the wall at shoulder height, keeping your elbows bent slightly.

Step 2: Slowly lift one leg straight up behind you, keeping your body still.

Step 3: Continue the movement, lowering the leg back down to the start position. Repeat, alternating legs.

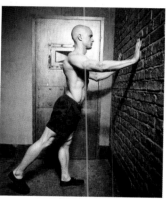

Tip: As a variation this exercise can be performed lying flat on your front and lifting your leg straight up behind or with your leg bent.

DOWN DOG WITH LEG LIFT

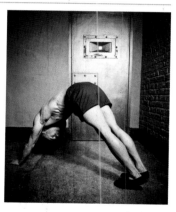

Target Muscle Groups
Primary: Gluteals
Secondary: Hamstrings, Abdominals, Deltoids

Step 1: Face downwards, with your hands on the floor, shoulder-width apart. Place your legs straight out behind you, with your feet together and your hips raised.

Step 2: Engage your abdominals and tighten your glutes. Extend one leg up high behind you.

Step 3: Continue the movement, lowering your leg back down to the floor. Repeat, raising your opposite leg up.

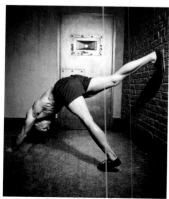

LEGS

KNEELING SQUAT

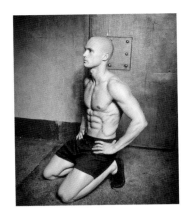

Target Muscle Groups
Primary: Quadriceps, Gluteals
Secondary: Hamstrings

Step 1: Kneel on the floor with your hands on your hips. Squeeze your shoulder blades together.

Step 2: Sit back and down until your glutes make contact with your calves.

Step 3: Continue the movement, raising back up and pushing your hips forward.

Tip: You may want to put something under your knees for support.

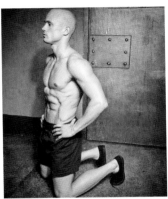

FALLING TOWER

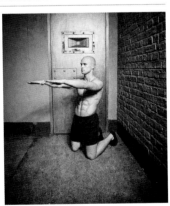

Target Muscle Groups
Primary: Quadriceps, Gluteals
Secondary: Hamstrings

Step 1: Kneel on the floor with your body upright and hands extended straight out in front of your chest, at shoulder height for balance.

Step 2: Looking straight ahead, keep your abdominals engaged and no bend at the hips. Slowly hinge at the knees and lean backwards, maintaining a straight back.

Step 3: Continue the movement, slowly raising your upper body back up to the start position.

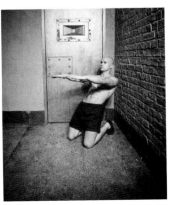

LEGS

CELL WORKOUT

KNEELING STEP UP

Target Muscle Groups
Primary: Quadriceps, Gluteals
Secondary: Hamstrings

Step 1: Kneel on the floor with your body upright and hands on your hips.

Step 2: Raise one foot to place it flat on the floor, then push up into a standing position.

Step 3: Continue the movement, kneeling back down to the starting position. Repeat, alternating legs.

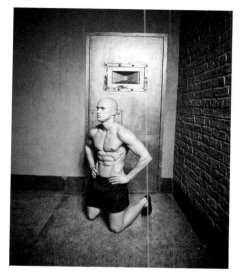

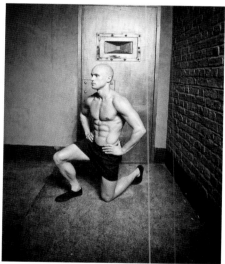

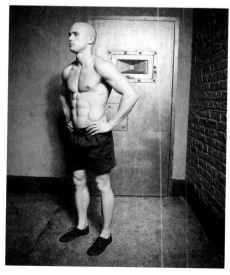

LEGS

KNEELING LEG LIFT

Target Muscle Groups
Primary: Gluteals
Secondary: Hamstrings, Quadriceps, Erector Spinae, Abdominals

Step 1: Kneel on all fours, hands directly under your shoulders, fingers pointing forwards and your knees under your hips. Extend one leg straight behind you and point your toes.

Step 2: Keep your eyes fixed on the floor and engage your abdominals. Slowly lift the extended leg up behind you.

Step 3: Continue the movement, lowering your leg back down, lightly touching your toes on the floor and immediately raise your leg back up. Repeat, alternating legs.

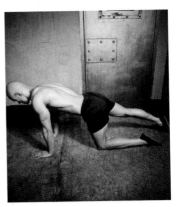

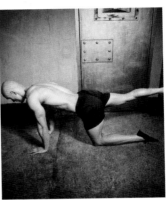

KNEELING LEG EXTENSION

Target Muscle Groups
Primary: Gluteals
Secondary: Hamstrings, Quadriceps, Erector Spinae, Abdominals

Step 1: Kneel on all fours, hands directly under your shoulders, elbows slightly bent and knees under your hips. Engage your abdominals and keep your back in a neutral position throughout the exercise.

Step 2: Keep your eyes fixed on the floor. Extend one leg straight behind you, so that it is inline with your hips. Try to keep your hips and shoulders still. Maintain a straight line with your body from your head to the heel of your extended leg.

Step 3: Continue the movement, slowly bringing your knee back in to the start position. Repeat, alternating legs.

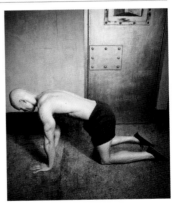

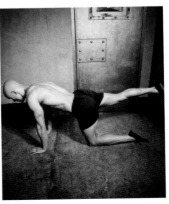

KNEELING BENT KNEE HEEL RAISE

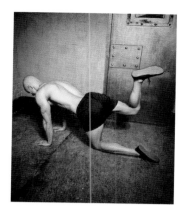

Target Muscle Groups

Primary: Gluteals

Secondary: Hamstrings, Quadriceps, Erector Spinae, Abdominals

Step 1: Kneel on all fours, hands directly under your shoulders, fingers pointing forwards and your knees under your hips. Lift one leg up behind so that it is level with your hips, with your knee bent to a 90-degree angle.

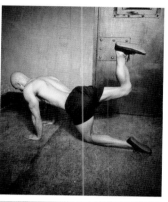

Step 2: Keep your eyes fixed on the floor. Engage your abdominals and push your heel up towards the ceiling. Keep your hips and shoulders in a square position to the floor during the exercise.

Step 3: Continue the movement, lowering your leg back down to the start position. Repeat, alternating legs.

Tip: Aim to keep your feet and heels facing in the same direction as you raise up, to avoid rotating your heels inwards.

KNEELING HYDRANT

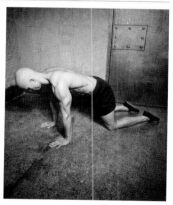

Target Muscle Groups

Primary: Gluteals

Secondary: Hamstrings, Quadriceps, Erector Spinae, Abdominals

Step 1: Kneel on all fours, hands directly under your shoulders, fingers pointing forwards and your knees under your hips.

Step 2: Keep your eyes fixed on the floor. Engage your abdominals and maintain your back in a straight line. Slowly raise one leg out to the side, with your knee bent to a 90-degree angle and your foot flexed. Keep your hips and shoulders in a square position to the floor as you lift your leg up.

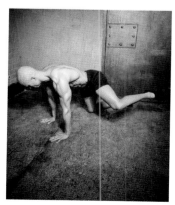

Step 3: Continue the movement, lowering your leg back down to the start position. Repeat, alternating legs.

KNEELING HYDRANT WITH LEG EXTENSION

Target Muscle Groups
Primary: Gluteals, Quadriceps
Secondary: Abdominals, Deltoids, Quadriceps

Step 1: Kneel on all fours, hands directly under your shoulders, fingers pointing forwards and your knees under your hips.

Step 2: Keep your eyes fixed on the floor. Engage your abdominals and maintain your back in a straight line. Slowly lift one leg out to the side, with your knee bent to a 90-degree angle and your foot flexed. Keep your hips and shoulders in a square position to the floor as you lift your leg up.

Step 3: Extend your leg out straight behind you.

Step 4: Continue the movement, slowly tucking your knee back in to the start position. Repeat, alternating legs.

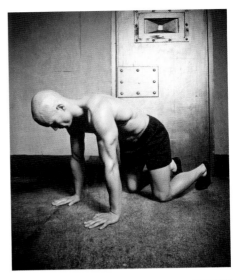
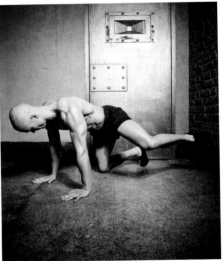
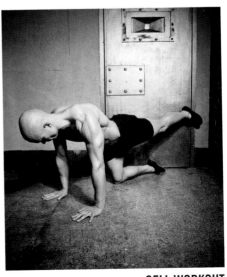

LEGS

KNEELING HYDRANT WITH SIDE KICK

Target Muscle Groups
Primary: Gluteals, Quadriceps
Secondary: Hamstrings, Erector Spinae, Abdominals

Step 1: Kneel on all fours, hands directly under your shoulders, fingers pointing forwards and your knees under your hips.

Step 2: Keep your eyes fixed on the floor. Engage your abdominals and maintain your back in a straight line. Slowly lift one leg out to the side, with your knee bent to a 90-degree angle and your foot flexed. Keep your hips and shoulders in a square position to the floor as you lift your leg up.

Step 3: Straighten the leg to extend it out to the side, then return to the bent-knee position.

Step 4: Continue the movement, reversing the action back down to the start position. Repeat, alternating legs.

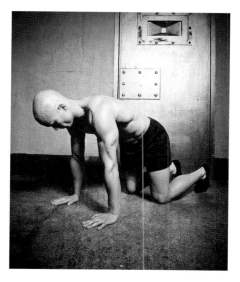

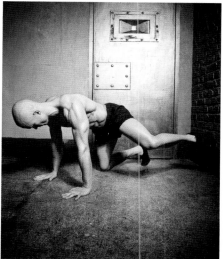

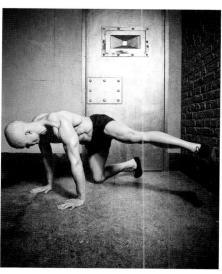

LEGS

GLUTE BRIDGE

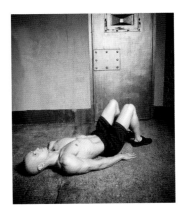

Target Muscle Groups
Primary: Gluteals
Secondary: Hamstrings, Erector Spinae

Step 1: Lie on your back, with your arms straight by your sides and palms down. Bend your knees and place your feet flat on the floor, hip-width apart.

Step 2: Engage your glutes and push through your heels to raise your pelvis upwards to form a straight line with your knees, hips and shoulders.

Step 3: Continue the movement, slowly uncurling your spine to lower back down to the floor.

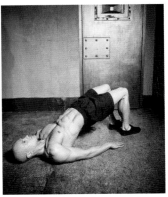

Tip: Avoid using your hands to help you push up.

GLUTE BRIDGE WITH RESTING BENT LEG

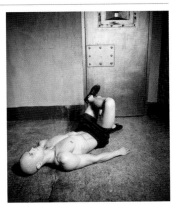

Target Muscle Groups
Primary: Gluteals
Secondary: Hamstrings, Erector Spinae

Step 1: Lie on your back with both legs bent and feet flat on the floor. Bend one leg and place the foot on the knee of the supporting leg. Place your arms by your sides and palms down.

Step 2: Engage your glutes and push through your heel to raise your pelvis upwards to form a straight line with your knees, hips and shoulders.

Step 3: Continue the movement, slowly uncurling your spine to lower back down to the floor. Repeat, alternating legs.

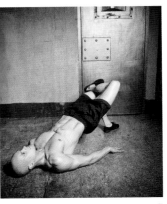

GLUTE BRIDGE WITH BENT KNEE LIFT

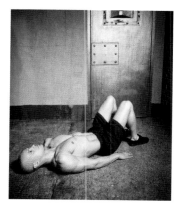

Target Muscle Groups
Primary: Gluteals, Quadriceps
Secondary: Hamstrings, Erector Spinae, Abdominals

Step 1: Lie on your back with both legs bent and feet flat on the floor, hip-width apart. Place your arms by your sides and palms down.

Step 2: Engage your glutes and push through your heels to raise your pelvis upwards to form a straight line with your knees, hips and shoulders. At the same time raise one knee up towards the ceiling.

Step 3: Continue the movement, slowly uncurling your spine to lower back down to the floor. Repeat, alternating legs.

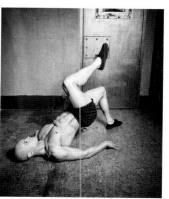

GLUTE BRIDGE WITH LOW STRAIGHT LEG LIFT

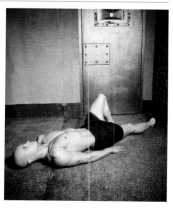

Target Muscle Groups
Primary: Gluteals, Quadriceps
Secondary: Hamstrings, Erector Spinae, Abdominals

Step 1: Lie on your back, with your arms straight by your sides and palms down. Bend one knee and place your foot flat on the floor. Extend the other leg out straight.

Step 2: Push through your heels to raise your pelvis upwards to form a straight line with your knees, hips and shoulders. At the same time raise the extended leg until your knees are inline with each other.

Step 3: Continue the movement, slowly uncurling your spine to lower back down to the floor. Repeat, alternating legs.

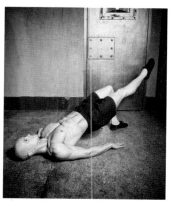

LEGS

GLUTE BRIDGE WITH HIGH STRAIGHT LEG LIFT

Target Muscle Groups
Primary: Gluteals, Quadriceps
Secondary: Hamstrings, Erector Spinae, Abdominals

Step 1: Lie on your back, with your arms straight by your sides and palms down. Bend one knee and place your foot flat on the floor. Extend the other leg out straight.

Step 2: Push through your heels to raise your pelvis upwards to form a straight line with your knees, hips and shoulders. At the same time raise the extended leg until your knees are inline with each other. Pause then lift the extended leg up higher towards the ceiling.

Step 3: Continue the movement, slowly uncurl your spine to lower back down to the floor. Repeat, alternating legs.

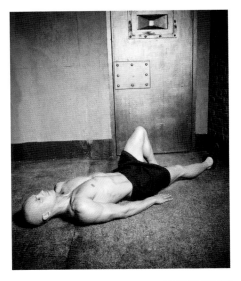

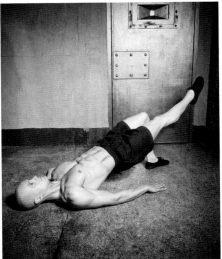

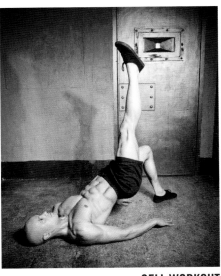

REVERSE TABLE TOP

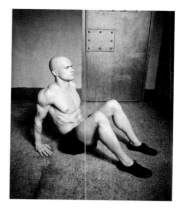

Target Muscle Groups
Primary: Gluteals, Hamstrings, Erector Spinae
Secondary: Deltoids, Triceps, Quadriceps

Step 1: Sit on the floor with knees bent and your feet flat in front of you. Place your hands underneath your shoulders so that your fingertips point towards your hips and your elbows point behind you.

Step 2: Engage your glutes, raise your hips up towards the ceiling to come to the upwards-facing tabletop position. Maintain your shoulders, hips, and knees in a straight line. Your shoulders should be directly over the top of your wrists.

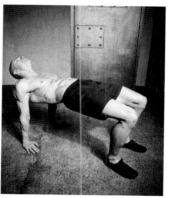

Step 3: Continue the movement, slowly uncurl your spine to lower back down to the start position.

REVERSE TABLE TOP WITH STRAIGHT LEG LIFT

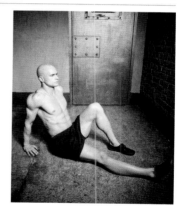

Target Muscle Groups
Primary: Gluteals, Hamstrings, Erector Spinae, Quadriceps
Secondary: Deltoids, Triceps, Abdominals

Step 1: Sit on the floor with knees bent and your feet flat in front of you. Extend your other leg out in front. Place your hands underneath your shoulders so that your fingertips point towards your hips and your elbows point behind you.

Step 2: Engage your glutes, raise your hips up towards the ceiling and lift the extended leg straight out so that your knees are in line with each other. Maintain your shoulders, hips, and knees in a straight line. Your shoulders should be directly above your wrists.

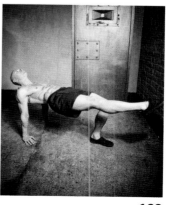

Step 3: Continue the movement, slowly uncurl your spine to lower back down to the start position.

SEATED STRAIGHT LEG LIFT

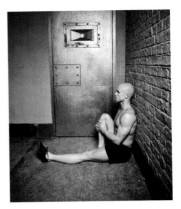

Target Muscle Groups
Primary: Quadriceps
Secondary: Hamstrings, Abdominals

Step 1: Sit upright on the floor with your back against a wall. Bend one leg and hold it in close to your chest. Extend the other leg straight out in front, with your foot flexed and toes pointing up.

Step 2: Engage your abdominals. Raise the extended leg off the floor a few inches.

Step 3: Continue the movement, lowering the leg touching the floor lightly. Repeat, then alternate legs.

Tips: By sitting upright, you limit your range of motion and your core will engage to keep your torso straight while lifting and lowering the leg.

This move is excellent for strengthening the quads and giving your knee joints more support.

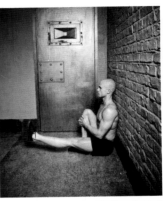

SEATED STRAIGHT LEG SWEEP

Target Muscle Groups
Primary: Quadriceps, Adductors
Secondary: Hamstrings, Abdominals

Step 1: Sit upright on the floor with your back against a wall. Bend one leg and hold it in close to your chest. Extend the other leg out straight in front, with your foot flexed and toes pointing up.

Step 2: Engage your abdominals. Raise the extended leg off the floor a few inches, then take it out to the side to a 45-degree angle.

Step 3: Continue the movement, returning you leg back to the center and lowering the leg, touching the floor lightly. Repeat, then alternate legs.

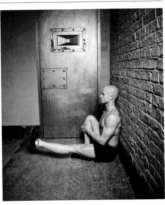

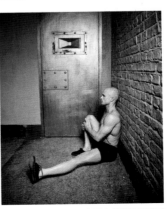

SIDE LYING LEG LIFT WITH HEAD RESTING

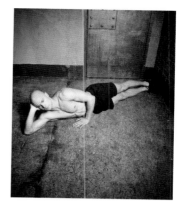

Target Muscle Groups
Primary: Gluteals, Quadriceps
Secondary:

Step 1: Lie on your side. Bend your supporting elbow and rest your head on your hand. Place your other hand in front for balance. Extend your legs out straight, one on top of each other.

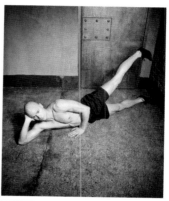

Step 2: Keeping your knees and toes pointing forward, slowly raise your upper leg towards the ceiling, until it is about 45-degrees off the floor.

Step 3: Continue the movement, slowly lower the upper leg back down. Repeat, then alternate on the opposite side.

SIDE LYING LEG LIFT WITH FOREARM RESTING

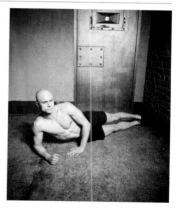

Target Muscle Groups
Primary: Gluteals, Quadriceps
Secondary:

Step 1: Lie on your side. Bend your supporting elbow to raise your upper body off the floor, resting on your forearm. Place your other hand in front for balance. Extend your legs out straight, one on top of each other.

Step 2: Keeping your knees and toes pointing forward, slowly raise your upper leg up towards the ceiling, keeping it straight, until it is about 45-degrees off the floor.

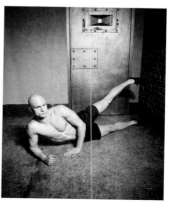

Step 3: Continue the movement, slowly lower the upper leg back down. Repeat, then alternate on the opposite side.

STANDING CALF RAISE

Target Muscle Groups

Primary: Gastrocnemius, Soleus

Secondary:

Step 1: Stand with your hands on your hips and feet hip-width apart.

Step 2: Engage your abdominals and raise your heels a few inches off the floor.

Step 3: Continue the movement, lowering your heels back down to the floor.

Tips: When doing any of the calf raise exercises, you may prefer to hold onto a wall or chair for support if needed.

For greater range of movement this exercise can be performed standing on the edge of a low raised platform to allow the heels to lower down further.

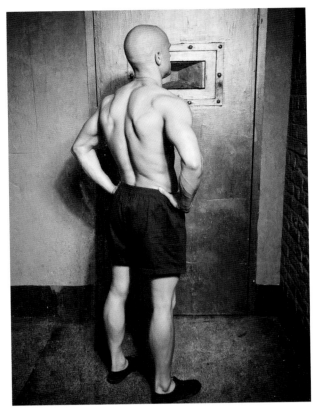

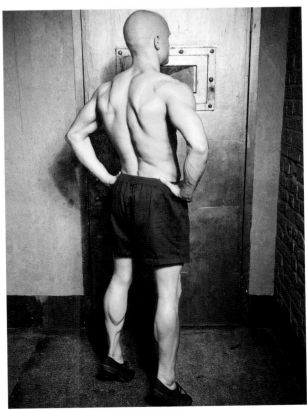

LEGS

172

INWARD CALF RAISE

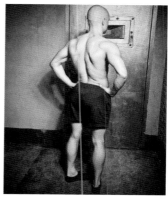

Target Muscle Groups
Primary: Gastrocnemius, Soleus
Secondary:

Step 1: Stand with your hands on your hips and feet hip-width apart, toes pointing inwards to a 45 degree angle.

Step 2: Engage your abdominals and raise your heels a few inches off the floor.

Step 3: Continue the movement, lowering your heels back down to the floor.

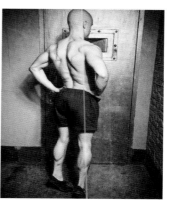

Tip: Aim to keep your feet and heels facing in the same direction as you raise up, to avoid rotating your heels inwards.

OUTWARD CALF RAISE

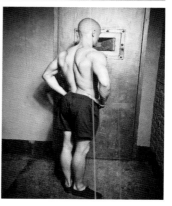

Target Muscle Groups
Primary: Gastrocnemius, Soleus
Secondary:

Step 1: Stand with your hands on your hips and feet hip-width apart, toes pointed out to a 45 degree angle.

Step 2: Engage your abdominals and raise your heels a few inches off the floor.

Step 3: Continue the movement, lowering your heels back down to the floor.

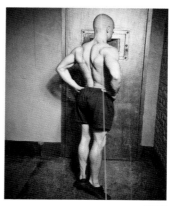

Tip: Aim to keep your feet and heels pointing in the same direction throughout the exercise.

LEGS

CALF RAISE WITH SINGLE LEG

Target Muscle Groups
Primary: Gastrocnemius, Soleus
Secondary: Abdominals

Step 1: Stand with your hands on your hips and feet hip-width apart.

Step 2: Engage your abdominals and lift one leg behind you. Raise the heel of the supporting foot a few inches off the floor.

Step 3: Continue the movement, lowering your heels back down to the floor. Repeat, then alternate by raising the other heel.

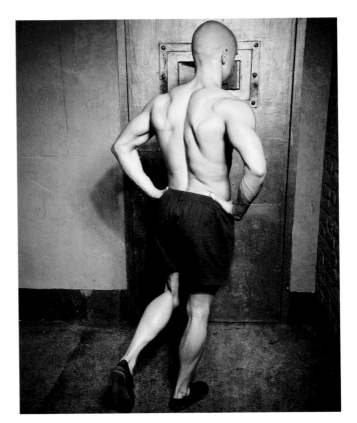

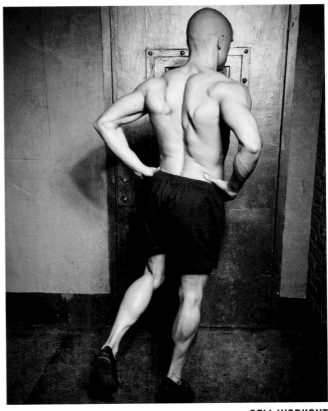

LEGS

GLUTE BRIDGE WITH CALF RAISE

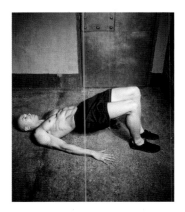

Target Muscle Groups
Primary: Gluteals, Gastrocnemius, Soleus
Secondary: Hamstrings, Erector Spinae

Step 1: Lie on your back with your arms straight by your sides and palms down. Bend your knees and place your feet flat on the floor, hip-width apart.

Step 2: Engage your glutes as you push through your heels to raise your pelvis upwards to form a straight line with your knees, hips and shoulders.

Step 3: Lift both heels up off the floor.

Step 4: Continue the movement, lowering your heels back to the floor.

Tips: If you are able to stay in the finish phase for a few seconds, it will also work your abdominal muscles. This exercise can also be performed using one leg at a time.

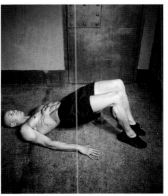

GLUTE BRIDGE WITH CALF RAISE TOE TAP

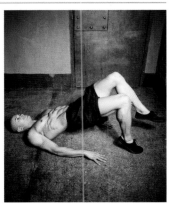

Target Muscle Groups
Primary: Gluteals, Gastrocnemius, Soleus
Secondary: Hamstrings, Erector Spinae, Abdominals

Step 1: Lie on your back with your arms straight by your sides and palms down. Bend your knees and place your feet flat on the floor, hip-width apart.

Step 2: Engage your glutes as you push through your heels to raise your pelvis upwards to form a straight line with your knees, hips and shoulders.

Step 3: Lift both heels up off the floor. With heels raised, lift one foot off the floor and then the other, in a marching action.

Step 4: Continue the movement, lowering your heels back to the floor.

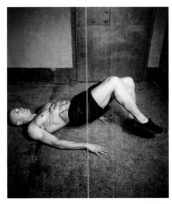

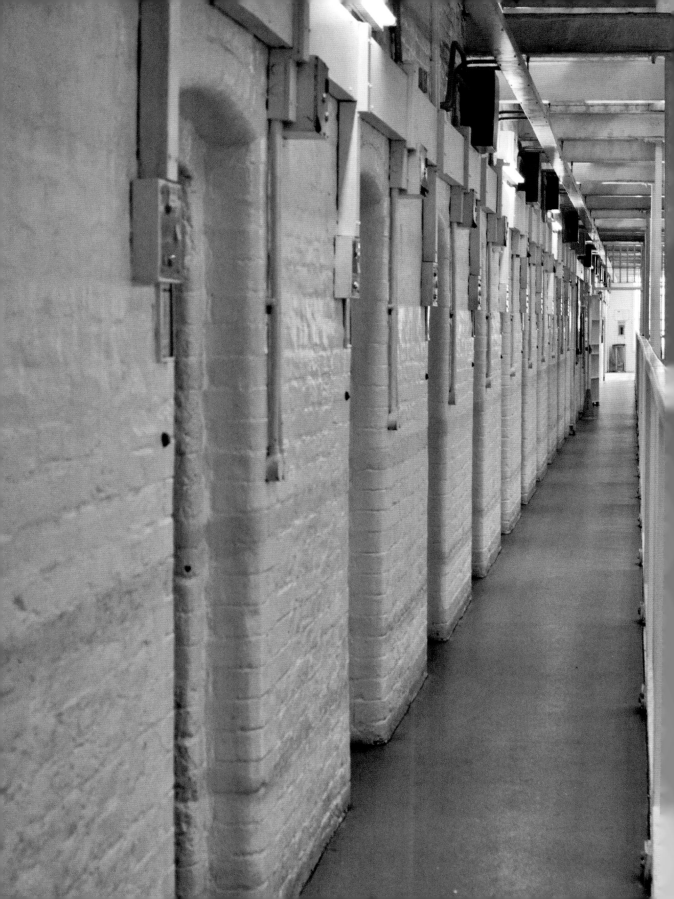

STATIC STRETCHES

Static stretching is a form of passive stretching. The stretches are performed by holding a limb yourself, against a wall or with the aid of a partner. This form of stretching will increase the muscle length and range of joint movement.

The purpose is to prevent the muscles tightening up and becoming sore, deliver oxygen and nutrients to the muscles and remove waste products.

The stretches should be performed after the muscles have been warmed up and is a important part of a cool down. The choice of stretch depends on what muscles have just been worked.

Static stretches will relax and lengthen the muscles that have been put under stress and help bring your body back toward a state of rest.

Static maintenance stretching is where the muscle is stretched to the end of its normal range and held without moving. These are short stretches, performed to help maintain the normal length of the muscle. During exercise the muscle becomes shorter and thicker as it repeatedly contracts. The maintenance stretch will return the muscle to its normal length.

Static development stretching is used to develop the length of the muscle fibres and increase the movement of a joint.

Performing static stretches at the appropriate time will improve and accelerate the recovery process after training.

Static stretching in an important part of the cool down to increase flexibility and prevent muscle soreness and injury.

LATERAL NECK FLEXION

Target Muscle Groups
Primary: Trapezius
Secondary:

Step 1: Stand with your arms by your sides.

Step 2: Keeping your head facing forwards and shoulders relaxed, slowly lower your ear down towards the shoulder closest to it. Hold the stretch.

Step 3: Release the stretch, gently return to the start position and repeat on the other side.

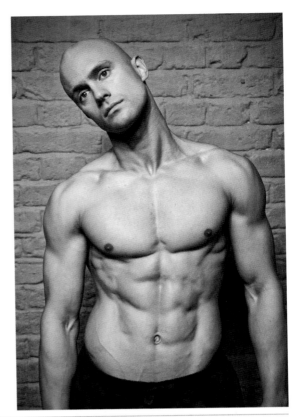

NECK ROTATION

Target Muscle Groups
Primary: Trapezius
Secondary:

Step 1: Stand with your arms by your sides.

Step 2: Relax your shoulders and keep them facing forwards. Keep your chin up as you slowly twist your neck and turn your head as far as you can in one direction. Hold the stretch.

Step 3: Release the stretch, gently return to the start position and repeat, turning your head to the other side.

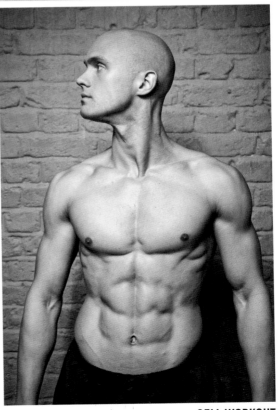

DIAGONAL NECK FLEXION

Target Muscle Groups
Primary: Trapezius, Rhomboids
Secondary:

Step 1: Stand with your arms by your sides.

Step 2: Relax your shoulders and gently lower your chin towards your chest then tilt your head to one side. Hold the stretch.

Step 3: Gently move your head back to the centre and then lift it back up to the start position. Repeat, lowering, then tilting your head to the other side.

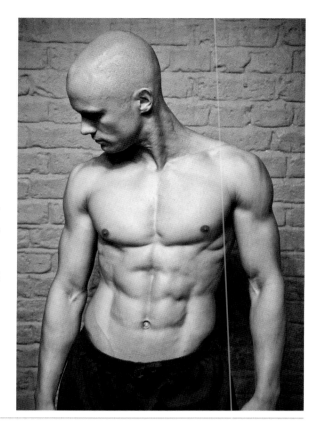

NECK FLEXION

Target Muscle Groups
Primary: Trapezius, Rhomboids
Secondary:

Step 1: Stand with your arms by your sides.

Step 2: Relax your shoulders and lower your chin gently towards your chest. Hold the stretch.

Step 3: With control, slowly raise your chin back up to the start position.

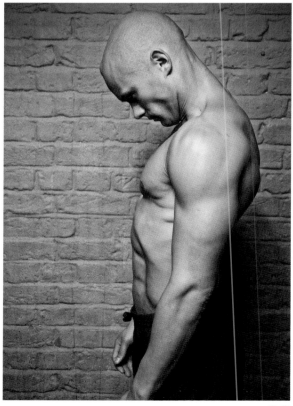

NECK EXTENSION

Target Muscle Groups
Primary: Trapezius
Secondary:

Step 1: Stand with your arms by your sides.

Step 2: Relax your shoulders and lift your head to look upwards, pointing your chin up, keeping your mouth closed. Hold the stretch.

Step 3: With control, slowly lower your chin back to the start position.

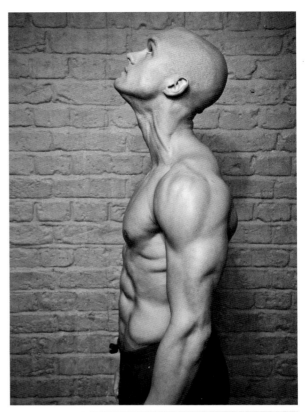

PARALLEL SINGLE ARM

Target Muscle Groups
Primary: Deltoids
Secondary:

Step 1: Stand with one arm across your chest. Bend the other arm and use it to pull the straight arm in towards your opposite shoulder.

Step 2: Hold and reach until you feel the stretch in your shoulder. Hold the stretch.

Step 3: Release the stretch, change arms and repeat.

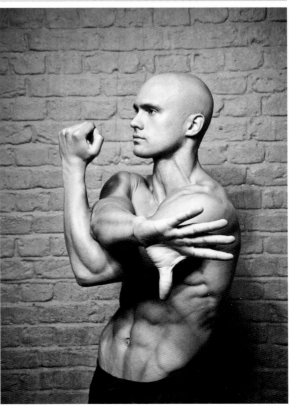

WRAP AROUND BACK

Target Muscle Groups
Primary: Rhomboids, Latissimus Dorsi, Deltoids
Secondary:

Step 1: Stand with your arms crossed over and wrap them around your shoulders.

Step 2: Slowly pull your shoulders back and hold the stretch at the lowest point you can reach.

Step 3: Hold the stretch, then release.

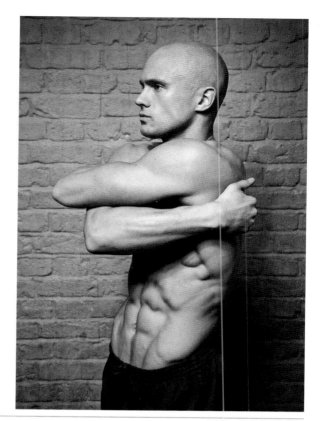

REVERSE SHOULDERS

Target Muscle Groups
Primary: Deltoids, Pectorals, Biceps
Secondary:

Step 1: Stand with your hands clasped behind your back and arms straight.

Step 2: Looking forwards and keeping your back still and straight, slowly lift your hands up behind you.

Step 3: Hold the stretch, then release.

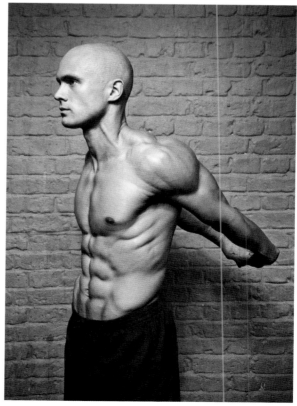

STATIC STRETCHES

EAGLE

Target Muscle Groups
Primary: Deltoids, Trapezius, Rhomboids
Secondary:

Step 1: Stand and bend both arms together, at 90-degree angles at shoulder-height. Keep your forearms crossed and hands together with your fingers pointing up towards the ceiling.

Step 2: Slowly raise your arms up as far as you can, keeping your arms together as you do so. Hold the stretch.

Step 3: Slowly release and gently lower your arms back to the start position.

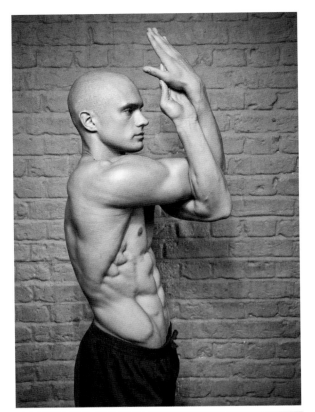

STRAIGHT ARM WALL CHEST

Target Muscle Groups
Primary: Pectorals, Deltoids, Biceps
Secondary:

Step 1: Stand next to a wall, with one arm extended slightly behind you at shoulder-height. Place your other arm by your side.

Step 2: Turn your body away from the wall. Hold the stretch.

Step 3: Release the stretch, change arms and repeat.

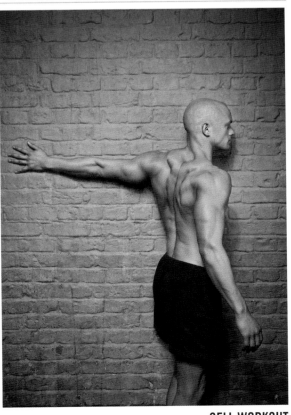

FORWARD REACHING UPPER BACK

Target Muscle Groups
Primary: Trapezius, Rhomboids
Secondary:

Step 1: Stand with your arms extended out in front of your chest, holding your hands together.

Step 2: Looking down, stretch your hands forwards and open up your shoulder-blades. Hold the stretch.

Step 3: Release the stretch and return to the start position.

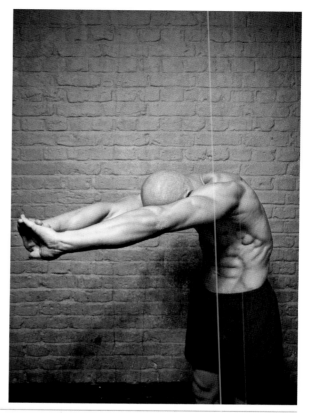

UPWARD REACHING LATISSIMUS DORSI

Target Muscle Groups
Primary: Latissimus Dorsi
Secondary:

Step 1: Stand with your arms extended straight up above your head, with your hands crossed over and fingers pointing upwards.

Step 2: Reach upwards towards the ceiling. Hold the stretch.

Step 3: Maintain the stretch before relaxing back to the start position.

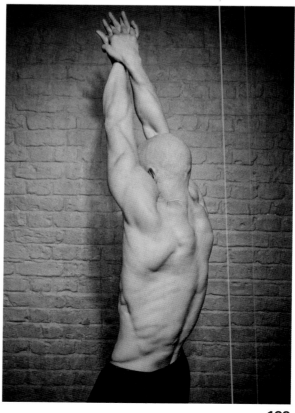

LATERAL REACHING LATISSIMUS DORSI

Target Muscle Groups
Primary: Latissimus Dorsi, Obliques Secondary:

Step 1: Stand with your feet shoulder-width apart and one arm extended straight above your head.

Step 2: Keeping your upper body straight, reach over your head with your extended arm, bending to the side.

Step 3: Hold the stretch before switching and reaching up and over with the other arm to bend to the other side.

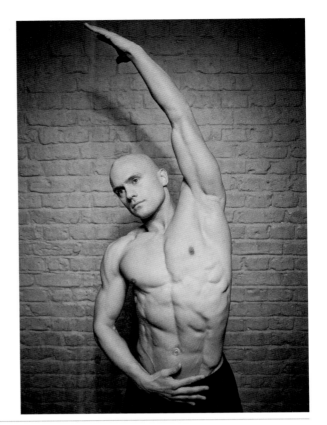

TORSO ROTATION

Target Muscle Groups
Primary: Obliques, Erector Spinae
Secondary:

Step 1: Stand with your feet shoulder-width apart. Extend your arms out to the sides, at shoulder-height, bend your elbows and place your hands on your shoulders.

Step 2: Looking straight ahead, rotate from your waist upwards round to one side. Hold the stretch then rotate back through the middle and then round to the other side.

Step 3: Continue rotating, keeping your arms raised.

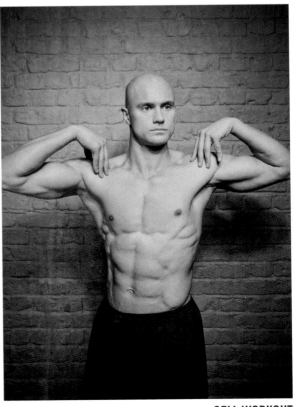

LEANING BACK ABDOMINALS

Target Muscle Groups
Primary: Abdominals
Secondary:

Step 1: Stand with your feet shoulder-width apart and place your hands on your lower back.

Step 2: Look up at the ceiling and gently lean back. Hold the stretch.

Step 3: Release the stretch and return to the start position.

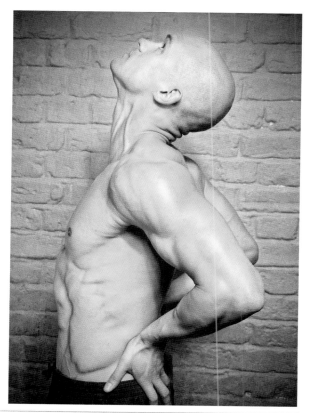

REACHING DOWN TRICEPS

Target Muscle Groups
Primary: Triceps, Latissimus Dorsi
Secondary:

Step 1: Bend both arms and reach behind your neck, with both elbows pointing upwards.

Step 2: Reach down your back with your hands. Hold the stretch.

Step 3: Release the stretch and return to the start position.

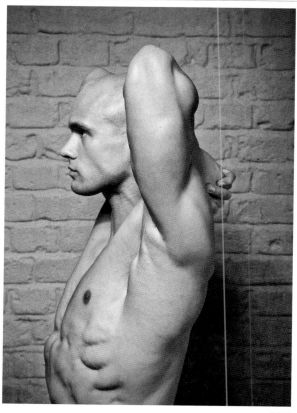

STATIC STRETCHES

SINGLE TRICEP

Target Muscle Groups
Primary: Triceps, Latissimus Dorsi
Secondary:

Step 1: Bend one arm and reach behind your neck, with your elbow pointing upwards.

Step 2: Reach across your head and hold onto your elbow with your other hand. Push your elbow downwards. Hold the stretch.

Step 3: Release the stretch and return to the start position. Repeat using the other arm.

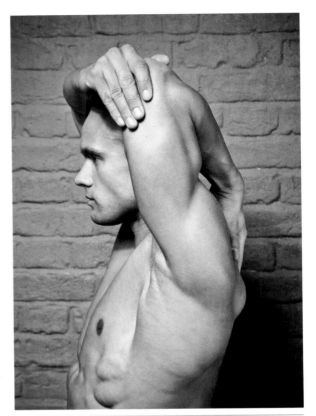

FORWARD REACHING PALMS OUT FOREARM

Target Muscle Groups
Primary: Rhomboids, Latissimus Dorsi, Trapezius
Secondary:

Step 1: Extend your arms straight out in front of your chest and interlock your fingers, with your palms facing outwards.

Step 2: Gently push your hands away from your body. Hold the stretch.

Step 3: Release the stretch and return to the start position.

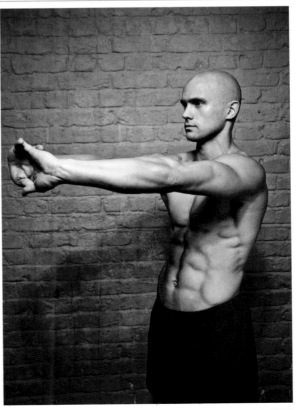

STANDING LEG RESTING GLUTES

Target Muscle Groups
Primary: Gluteals
Secondary:

Step 1: Stand next to a wall and hold on for support. Place your other hand on your hip. Bend your outside leg and place your ankle across the knee of your supporting leg.

Step 2: Slowly bend your supporting leg and lower down towards the floor. Hold the stretch.

Step 3: Release the stretch, then switch legs and repeat.

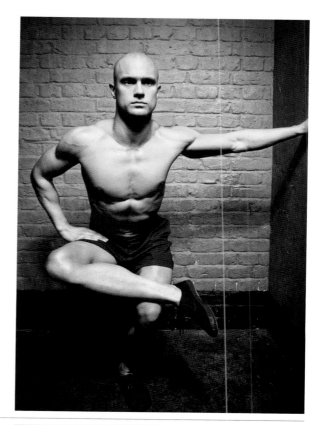

SEATED BENT OVER ERECTOR SPINAE

Target Muscle Groups
Primary: Erector Spinae, Adductors
Secondary:

Step 1: Sit on the floor, with your knees bent and the soles of your feet together.

Step 2: Lower your head and chest forwards, relaxing your back and neck. Hold the stretch.

Step 3: Release the stretch and return to the start position.

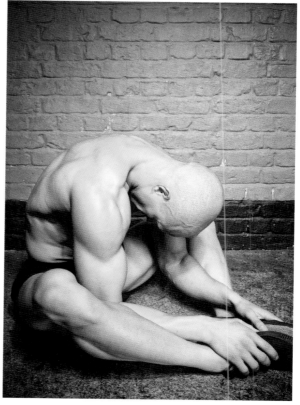

KNEE ACROSS TORSO ROTATION

Target Muscle Groups

Primary: Gluteals, Erector Spinae, Obliques

Secondary:

Step 1: Sit with one leg extended straight out in front and the other leg bent and crossed over your straight leg. Keep the foot of the bent leg flat on the floor.

Step 2: Put your opposite arm across your bent leg and your other hand behind you on the floor for support. Rotate your upper body and look back in the same direction as the hand that is behind.

Step 3: Hold the stretch then switch sides and repeat.

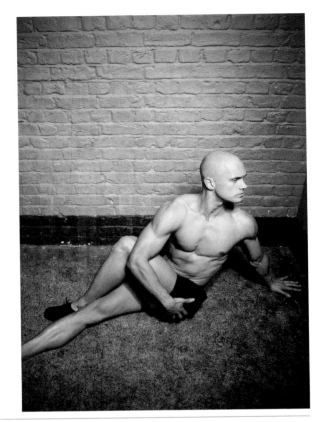

LYING LEG ACROSS

Target Muscle Groups

Primary: Gluteals, Obliques, Erector Spinae, Pectorals

Secondary:

Step 1: Lie on your back, with your legs extended straight out in front and your arms straight out to the sides at shoulder-height.

Step 2: Keeping your shoulders on the floor, lift one leg, bend the knee and place it across and down on the floor. Press onto the bent knee with your opposite hand to increase the stretch. Hold the stretch.

Step 3: Release the stretch, then switch legs and repeat, pressing onto the other knee.

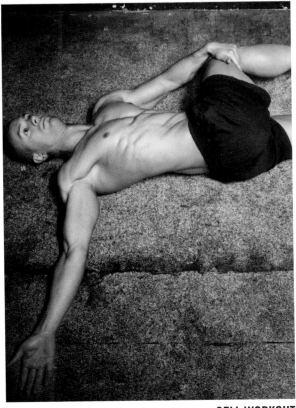

LYING SINGLE KNEE TO CHEST

Target Muscle Groups
Primary: Gluteals, Erector Spinae
Secondary:

Step 1: Lie on your back with one leg extended and flat on the floor. Bend the other leg towards your chest and hold at the knee.

Step 2: Without raising your upper body or lifting your head, gently pull your knee in towards your chest. Hold the stretch.

Step 3: Release the stretch, then switch legs and repeat.

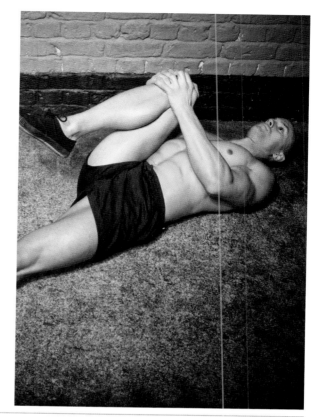

LYING LEG RESTING GLUTES

Target Muscle Groups
Primary: Gluteals
Secondary:

Step 1: Lie on your back, with one leg bent and place the other foot across your bent knee. Reach your hands through your legs and clasp them around your thigh.

Step 2: Gently pull your thigh towards your chest. Hold the stretch.

Step 3: Release the stretch, then switch legs and repeat.

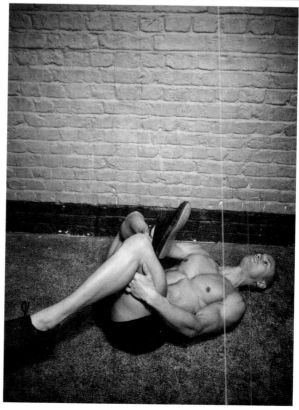

KNEELING QUADRICEPS

Target Muscle Groups
Primary: Gluteals
Secondary:

Step 1: Place one knee on the floor and your other foot flat on the floor in front with your leg bent at 90-degree angle, with your knee directly over your ankle and your thigh parallel to the floor. Place your hands on your hips.

Step 2: Look straight ahead and, maintaining a straight back, gently push your hips forwards. Hold the stretch.

Step 3: Release the stretch, then switch legs and repeat.

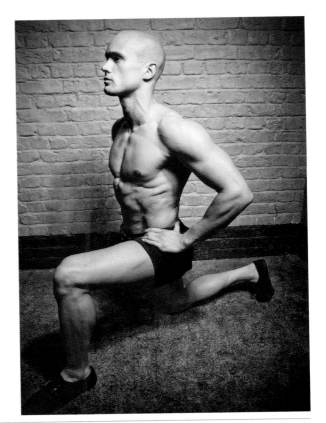

STANDING QUADRICEPS

Target Muscle Groups
Primary: Quadriceps
Secondary:

Step 1: Stand next to a wall and hold on for support. With your knees close together, use your other hand to hold one foot up behind your buttocks.

Step 2: Look straight ahead and, maintaining a straight back, push your hips forwards slightly. Hold the stretch.

Step 3: Release the stretch, then switch legs and repeat.

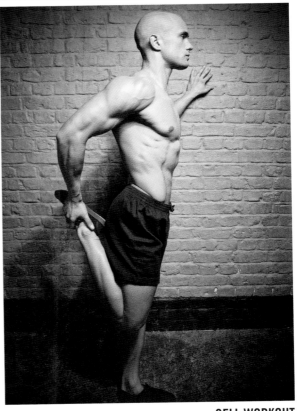

LEANING BACK QUADRICEPS

Target Muscle Groups
Primary: Quadriceps
Secondary:

Step 1: Sit on the floor with one leg bent under your buttocks and the other leg bent with foot flat on the floor. Place your hands on the floor behind you.

Step 2: Slowly lean backwards until you feel the stretch in your quad muscle. Hold the stretch.

Step 3: Release the stretch, then switch legs and repeat.

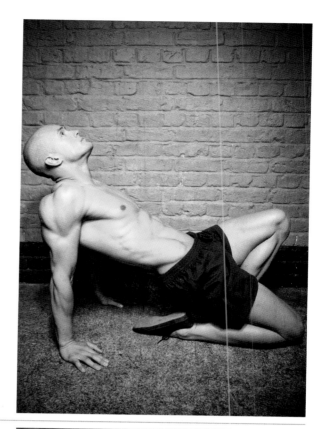

LYING BENT KNEE HAMSTRINGS

Target Muscle Groups
Primary: Hamstrings, Gluteals
Secondary:

Step 1: Lie on your back, with one leg bent and your foot flat on the floor. Raise the other leg, holding it with both hands behind the knee.

Step 2: Without raising your upper body, slowly pull your raised leg, with bent knee, in towards your chest. Hold the stretch.

Step 3: Release the stretch, then switch legs and repeat.

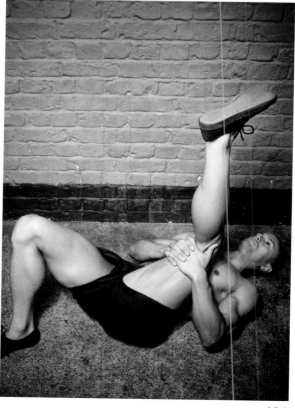

STATIC STRETCHES

SEATED KNEES OUT ADDUCTORS

Target Muscle Groups
Primary: Adductors
Secondary:

Step 1: Sit upright, with the soles of your feet together. Hold onto your ankles and rest your elbows on your knees.

Step 2: Looking straight ahead and maintaining a straight back, push down with your elbows to lower your knees towards the floor. Hold the stretch.

Step 3: Gently release the stretch and return to the start position.

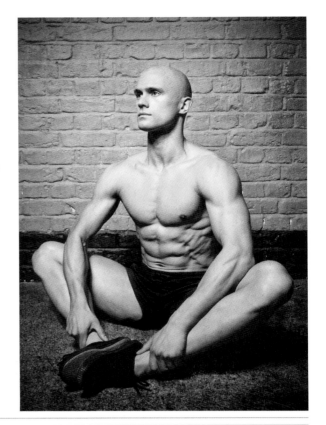

LATERAL LUNGE ADDUCTORS

Target Muscle Groups
Primary: Adductors
Secondary:

Step 1: Stand with your feet wide apart, with one leg straight and the other leg bent, toes pointing out slightly to the sides. Place your hands on your hips.

Step 2: Looking straight ahead and maintaining a straight back, lower down towards the floor so you can feel the extension in your adductor muscle. Hold the stretch.

Step 3: Release the stretch, then switch legs and repeat.

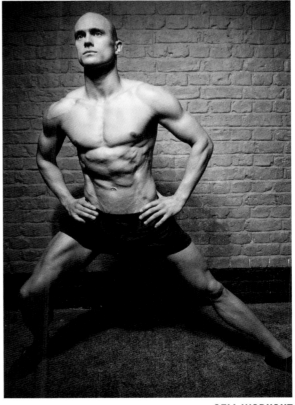

TOE UP WALL CALVES

Target Muscle Groups
Primary: Gastrocnemius, Soleus
Secondary:

Step 1: Stand facing a wall, holding on for support if needed. Place the toes of one foot against the wall.

Step 2: Keeping your leg straight, lean towards your toes so you can feel the extension in your calf muscle. Hold the stretch.

Step 3: Release the stretch, then switch legs and repeat.

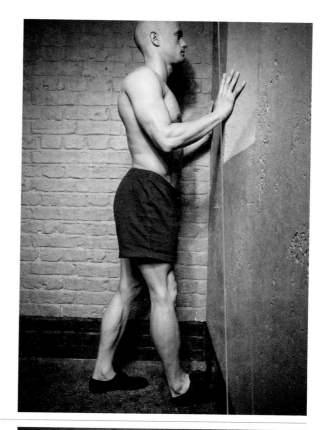

KNEELING HEEL DOWN ACHILLES

Target Muscle Groups
Primary: Gastrocnemius, Soleus
Secondary:

Step 1: Kneel with one leg on the floor and your other leg bent with your foot flat on the floor. Place your hands flat on the floor in front on you.

Step 2: Gently move your hands forward to stretch the area below your calf. Hold the stretch.

Step 3: Release the stretch, then switch legs and repeat.

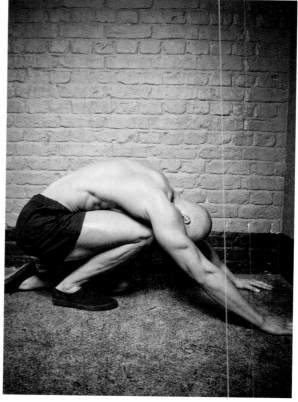

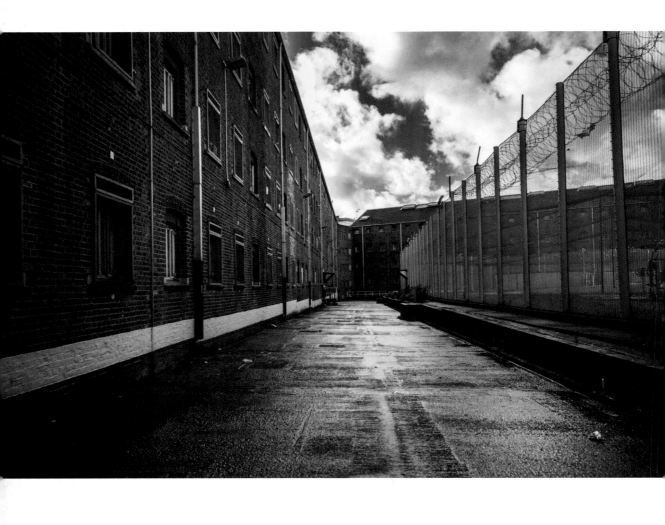

RELAXATION

Relaxation technique or training, can be any method or activity that helps a person to relax the body, calm the mind and as a result reduce anxiety, stress or anger. Relaxation is also thought to be beneficial to physical health and improving sleep quality.

After exercise, it will give the body the chance to regroup and rest. Relaxation should be performed after you have cooled down and stretched, before you go to bed, or whenever you feel the need.

Make sure you are comfortable and wear loose clothing.

Any relaxation starts by focusing on your breathing.

To control your breathing; take slow, deep breaths, slowly in through your nose and out through your mouth, in a steady rhythm, without forcing the breath.

Relax your shoulders and upper chest muscles when you breathe so you are mainly using your diaphragm.

As you exhale, imagine all the tension and negative energy slowly moving out of your body. If you notice any areas where you feel tension, relax them as you exhale. Breathing in this way will help to increase your mind-body awareness and concentrate your energy on muscle relaxation.

Feel your muscles relaxing and growing heavier.

Work your way through your entire body, focusing on relaxing one muscle group at a time, starting at the bottom and working up.

Basic relaxation techniques are not difficult but take practice. Everybody reacts differently so experiment to find what techniques work for you. You may find it helpful to listen to music that creates a peaceful atmosphere. Start with 10 minutes a day and increase as you get used to it.

Being able to spend time practising relaxation will quiet your mind, boost your energy levels and promote positive thoughts.

CORPSE POSE (SAVASANA)

This simple pose brings complete relaxation, with an awareness of your breath. It can be performed to give your muscles a rest and before sleep.

Step 1: Lie on your back. Allow your feet to fall outwards and place your arms by your sides, not too close to your body, with palms facing up.

Step 2: Relax your whole body, including the face so that your body feels heavy. Breathe naturally without forcing it.

Step 3: Inhale and hold your breath. At the same time stretch yourself out, so that your whole body is tense. Hold for a few seconds.

Step 4: Exhale and relax your body. When you are ready to come out of your relaxation, begin by breathing more deeply. Move your fingers and toes as you awaken your body.

Step 5: Bring your knees into your chest and roll over to one side, keeping your eyes closed.

Step 6: Slowly bring yourself up into a sitting position.

Tips: This is a resting pose, stay in the present and remain aware during your time of relaxation.

As a variation, bend at the knees so your feet are flat to the floor, hip-width apart.

Relax your knees inwards so they are touching.

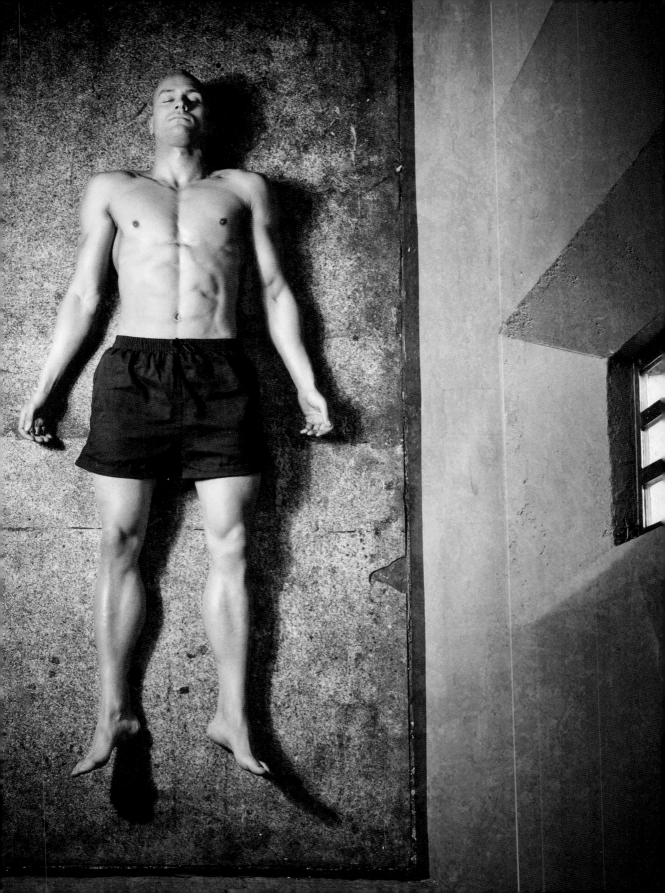

LEGS UP THE WALL POSE (VIPARITA KARANI)

This pose can help relieve aching feet, legs and lower back.

Step 1: Sit with one side against the wall. Lower your body down and turn so that you place your back on the floor and bring your legs straight up onto the wall.

Step 2: Shift your weight forwards until your glutes are close to the wall. Place your arms at your sides, palms facing up.

Step 3: Close your eyes. Breathe gently and remain aware.

Step 4: When you are ready to come out of your relaxation, slowly push yourself away from the wall and slide your legs down to the side. Use your hands to help press yourself up into a seated position.

Tips: It is important to feel comfortable and relaxed throughout the duration of the pose.

Obtain medical advice if you suffer from high or low blood presssure or any other condition.

If you have a sore neck, place a folded towel under it or pillow under your head. if your back is not comfortable adjust your body so that you are further away from the wall.

To stretch your inner thighs and groin, let your legs fall outwards to form a 'V' shape.

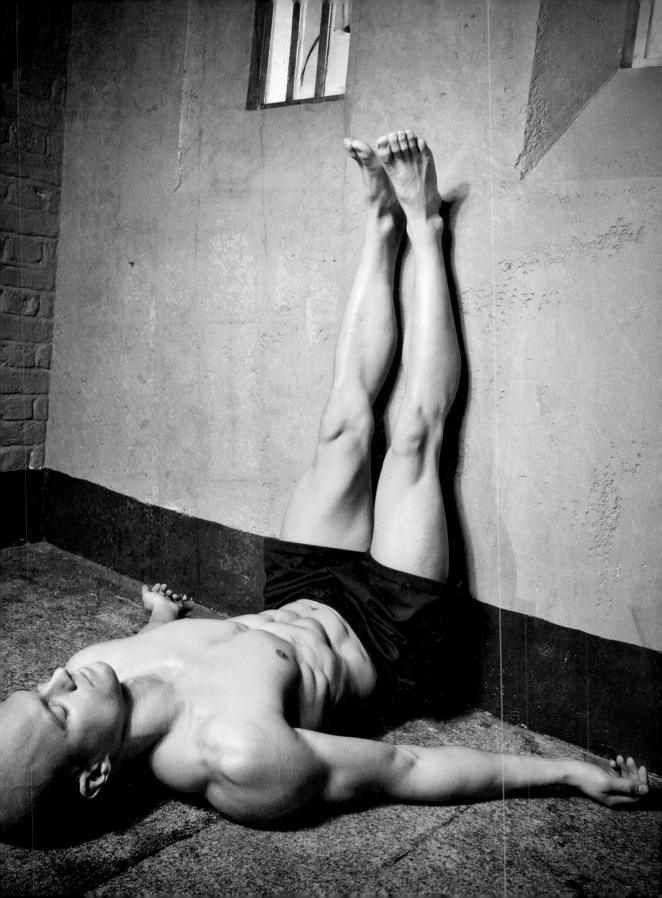

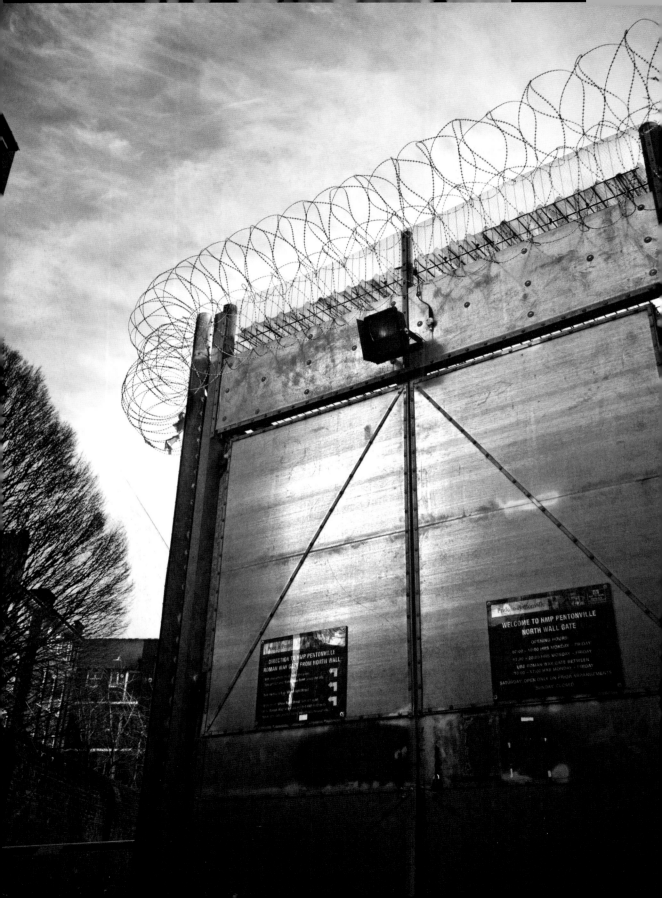

MEDITATION

Meditation is the art of focusing the mind. People meditate for different reasons and it can help in different ways; increase concentration, promote inner calm and peace, lessen anxiety, solve problems and improve sleep.

Meditation practice will be different for each person, but the basics of meditation are relaxation and breathing. Some people find that first thing in the morning is a good time to meditate but choose any time that works for you.

SIMPLE MEDITATION

Sit quietly, with legs crossed, or out straight, or in a chair, however is comfortable for you. Sit on the edge of a folded towel if necessary.

Place your hands on your knees or by your sides, with palms facing up.

Face forwards, with head up and spine straight.

Closing your eyes may make it easier to concentrate, but leave them open if you prefer. Relax your face, jaw and tongue.

Turn your attention inwards and concentrate on your breathing. Breathe in through the nose and out through the mouth. Breathe deeply from the diaphragm, not shallow breathing, until you feel calm.

Think about all your body parts, starting with your feet and work your way up. Focus on one point at a time.

If you find it hard to concentrate and you feel distractions creeping in, focus back on your breathing – in and out.

When you are ready to come out of meditation, sit still and quietly for a while before standing up slowly.

Begin with short sessions, this maybe for a few minutes at first, but 10 minutes a day increasing to 20 minutes is a good starting point.

Meditation is an active process that focuses the mind on the internal, away from your everyday thoughts. With practice and perseverance you will benefit from taking the time to be still and quiet the mind.

EASY POSE (SUKHASANA)

This pose creates the conditions for a relaxed body and alert mind; keeping the head and neck aligned with the spine, whilst maintaining a straight spine throughout the meditation session.

Step 1: Sit on the edge of a folded up towel or on the floor. Extend your legs straight out in front of your body and sit up straight.

Step 2: Cross your legs in front of you, with your knees out wide. Balance your weight evenly across your sit bones*. Relax your feet and thighs. Place your hands on your knees, palms up.

Step 3: Lengthen your spine, with your neck and head straight. Look straight ahead.

Step 4: Hold the position for the duration of your meditation.

*Tips: * the sit bones refer to the bones that are at the bottom of the pelvis that you sit on.*

If you have a knee injury or are not able to sit comfortably with your legs crossed, adopt a position that is comfortable for you.

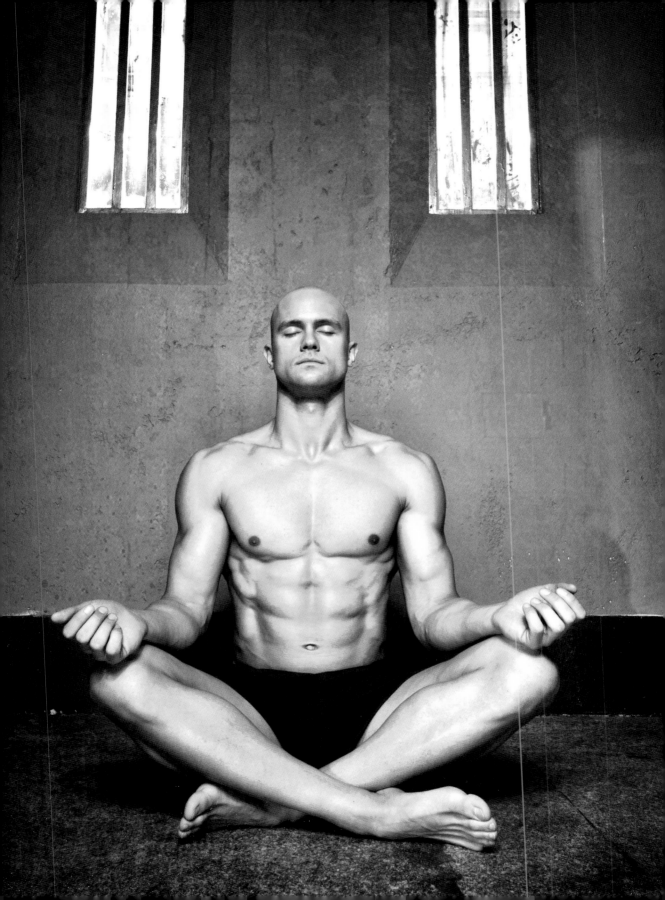

THE CELL WORKOUT

This is a 10 week program based on my version of the 'Cell Workout', aimed to give you a starting point, by having something to follow. It is made up of the first 6 weeks bodyweight training, followed by 4 weeks cardio.

The exercises selected offer a natural progression in difficulty each week. If you find that some are too easy and are not giving enough stimulus to the muscles or if you find any too hard to perform, then change the exercises to suit your personal needs.

Rest days have been included, with more rest days at the beginning of the program and less towards the end. If you are still aching the next day then adapt your program taking an additonal rest day or if you feel fine then drop out a rest day.

The workouts do not differ in structure and are suitbale for all levels of fitness. Follow the guidelines to differentiate between beginner, intermediate and advanced. But still these are only guidelines and the reps, sets and rest periods can be altered to suit your needs.

BODYWEIGHT TRAINING GUIDELINES (WEEKS 1-6)

Level	Reps	Sets	Rest	Duration (approx)
Beginner	10+	2	90 seconds	45 minutes
Intermediate	12+	3	60 seconds	60 minutes
Advanced	15+	3	30 seconds	45 minutes

With the 6 week bodyweight workouts you count the amount of reps for a set. Each set taking 30 seconds to complete on average.

CARDIOVASCULAR BODYWEIGHT TRAINING GUIDELINES (WEEKS 7-10)

Level	Set Duration	Sets	Rest	Duration (approx)
Beginner	30 seconds	3	30 seconds	20 minutes
Intermediate	45 seconds	3	30 seconds	30 minutes
Advanced	60 seconds	3	30 seconds	40 minutes

In the 4 week cardio workouts; on Tuesdays, Thursdays and Sundays, the rhythm session includes cardio bodyweight exercises. The sets are measured by duration as opposed to reps.

ISOMETRIC TRAINING GUIDELINES

Level	Set Duration
Beginner	30 seconds
Intermediate	60 seconds
Advanced	90 seconds

With isometric exercises like Plank, Side Plank, Wall Sit and Chest Squeeze, where it is not possible to count the reps, you will need to time the duration.

By using a stopwatch or seconds hand on a clock you will be able to time your training and rest periods. This will help keep your workout timings structured. To get an understanding of the exercises you are about to perform, read up on them before you begin. If you need to check any as you go along, refer back to the exercise page during your timed rest break.

A vital part of any workout is the warm up and cool down. The routines are included in full on pages 30-31. They are designed for all abilities and are suitable before and after the bodyweight and cardio workouts.

The time of day you train will play a part in the overall efficiency of the workout. Find a time of day that works for you. It is best to train in the morning after breakfast, allowing an hour and half after eating. This is when your energy is at its highest as you are fully rested after sleep.

Wear clothing that is comfortable and fits well, how many layers you wear will depend on the temperature you train in. Wear trainers that fit properly to help absorb impact and protect your joints.

Using an exercise mat when performing floor exercises will protect your elbows, knees, spine and tailbone.

Make sure you drink plenty of water to stay hydrated during the workout and throughout the day and also maintain a healthy and balanced diet.

Motivation is key, listening to high tempo music with a good beat will get you inspired and keep you motivated during your workout.

Following these tips and guidelines will help you get the most out of your training and get the body you want – **Inside & Out**.

WEEK 1 – FULL BODY

MONDAY

Exercise	Page
Squat	150
Glute Bridge	166
Standing Calf Raise	172
Hand Push	66
Supine Shoulder Elevation	74
I Formation with Arms In Front	71
Good Morning	96
Dorsal Raise with Fingers On Temples	106
Baby Cobra	100
Wall Press Up	80
Press Up On Knees	82
Chest Squeeze	89
Standing Crunch Pull	129
Crunch	118
Plank	138
Waist Pinch	131
Oblique Crunch	132
Side Plank	141

TUESDAY – Rest Day

WEDNESDAY

Exercise	Page
Squat	150
Glute Bridge	166
Standing Calf Raise	172
Hand Push	66
Supine Shoulder Elevation	74
I Formation with Arms In Front	71
Good Morning	96
Dorsal Raise with Fingers On Temples	106
Baby Cobra	100
Wall Press Up	80
Press Up On Knees	82
Chest Squeeze	89
Standing Crunch Pull	129
Crunch	118
Plank	138
Waist Pinch	131
Oblique Crunch	132
Side Plank	141

THURSDAY – Rest Day

FRIDAY

Exercise	Page
Close Hand Wall Press Up	81
Close Hand Press Up On Knees	82
Press Up	83
Forward Lunge	155
Glute Bridge with Resting Bent Leg	166
Kneeling Leg Lift	162
Shoulder Press Wall Slide	66
L Formation	72
Pike Shoulder Press	77
Good Morning with Arm By Sides	97
Scapular Retraction	114
Dorsal Raise with Fingers On Temples	102
Standing Oblique Twist	130
Oblique Crunch with Resting Bent Leg	134
Full Plank with Knee To Elbow	139
Crunch with Raised Bent Knees	119
Seated Knee Tuck with Single Leg	125
Full Plank	138

SATURDAY

Exercise	Page
Close Hand Wall Press Up	81
Close Hand Press Up On Knees	82
Press Up	83
Forward Lunge	155
Glute Bridge with Resting Bent Leg	166
Kneeling Leg Lift	162
Shoulder Press Wall Slide	66
L Formation	72
Pike Shoulder Press	77
Good Morning with Arms By Sides	97
Scapular Retraction	114
Dorsal Raise with Fingers On Temples	102
Standing Oblique Twist	130
Oblique Crunch with Resting Bent Leg	134
Full Plank with Knee To Elbow	139
Crunch with Raised Bent Knees	119
Seated Knee Tuck with Single Leg	125
Full Plank	138

SUNDAY – Rest Day

WEEK 2 – FULL BODY

MONDAY

Exercise	Page
Baby Cobra	100
Reverse Dorsal Raise with Single Leg	107
Full Dorsal Raise with Arms By Side	110
Press Up	83
Wide Hand Press Up	84
Single Arm Wall Press Up	81
Lateral Lunge	158
Side Lying Leg Lift with Head Resting	171
Glute Bridge with Calf Raise	175
Elbows In External Rotation	68
W Formation	73
Pike Shoulder Press	77
Crunch with Raised Bent Knees	119
Lying Knee Tuck with Single Leg	124
Full Plank with Single Knee Tuck	139
Oblique Crunch with Raised Bent Knees	133
Heel Tap	135
Side Plank with Straight Arm	141

WEDNESDAY

Exercise	Page
Baby Cobra	100
Reverse Dorsal Raise with Single Leg	107
Full Dorsal Raise with Arms By Side	110
Press Up	83
Wide Hand Press Up	84
Single Arm Wall Press Up	81
Lateral Lunge	158
Side Lying Leg Lift with Head Resting	171
Glute Bridge with Calf Raise	175
Elbows in External Rotation	68
W Formation	73
Pike Shoulder Press	77
Crunch with Raise Bent Knees	119
Lying Knee Tuck with Single Leg	124
Full Plank with Single Knee Tuck	139
Oblique Crunch with Raised Bent Knees	133
Heel Tap	135
Side Plank with Straight Arm	141

TUESDAY – Rest Day

THURSDAY

Exercise	Page
Supine Shoulder Flexion	70
I formation with Arms In Front	71
Pike Shoulder Press	77
Full Dorsal Raise with Arms By Side	110
Scapular Retraction	114
Superman	111
Wide Hand Press Up	84
Close Hand Press Up	84
Straight Arm Chest Squeeze	89
Prisoner Squat	152
Wall Sit	154
Seated Straight Leg Lift	170
Bicycle Crunch	137
Side Lying Oblique Crunch	134
Full Side Plank	146
Crunch with Vertical Straight Legs	119
High Scissors	128
Full Plank	138

SATURDAY

Exercise	Page
Supine Shoulder Flexion	70
I Formation with Arms In Front	71
Pike Shoulder Press	77
Full Dorsal Raise with Arms By Side	110
Scapular Retraction	114
Superman	111
Wide Hand Press Up	84
Close Hand Press Up	84
Straight Arm Chest Squeeze	89
Prisoner Squat	152
Wall Sit	154
Seated Straight Leg Lift	170
Bicycle Crunch	137
Side Lying Oblique Crunch	134
Full Side Plank	146
Crunch with Vertical Straight Legs	119
High Scissors	128
Full Plank	138

FRIDAY – Rest Day

SUNDAY – Rest Day

WEEK 3 – UPPER BODY & LOWER BODY

MONDAY – Upper

Exercise	Page
Press Up	83
Wide Hand Press Up	84
Close Hand Press Up	84
Straight Arm Chest Squeeze	89
Plyo Press Up	91
Good Morning with Arms By Side	97
Dorsal Raise with Hands Clasped Behind Back	104
Prone Heel Raise with Double Leg	108
Cobra	100
Cat Cow	98
Hand Grasp Pull	68
Y Formation	71
Full Plank Body Saw	75
Elbows In External Rotation	68
Pike Shoulder Press	77

TUESDAY – Lower

Exercise	Page
Squat With Rotation	152
Forward Lunge	155
Glute Bridge with Low Straight Leg Lift	167
Kneeling Leg Extension	162
Wall Sit	154
Seated Straight Leg Lift	170
Crunch with Raised Bent Knees	119
Single Leg Raise with Vertical Straight Leg	122
Shoulders Raised Lying Knee Tuck with Single Leg	124
Opposite Vertical Toe Reach	121
Double Leg Raise	123
Waist Pinch	131
Side Lying Oblique Crunch	134
Full Plank with Opposite Knee To Elbow	140
Side Plank with Straight Arm	141

WEDNESDAY – Rest Day

THURSDAY – Upper

Exercise	Page
Bent Arm Front Cross Over	67
Fast Hand Tap	74
Full Plank Body Saw	75
T Formation	72
Pike Shoulder Press	77
Press Up	83
Lateral Press Up	88
Close Hand Press Up	84
Plyo Press Up	91
Staggered Hand Press Up	86
Good Morning	96
Dorsal Raise with Rotation	102
Reverse Dorsal Raise with Double Leg	107
Superman	111
Dorsal Raise with Side Bend	103

FRIDAY – Lower

Exercise	Page
Oblique Crunch with Raised Bent Knees	133
Side Lying Oblique Crunch	134
Heel Tap	135
Side Plank with Torso Rotation	142
Prisoner Squat	152
Reverse Lunge	156
Seated Straight Leg Sweep	170
Kneeling Step Up	161
Glute Bridge with Bent Knee Lift	167
Inward Calf Raise	173
Crunch with Raised Bent Knees	119
Plank	138
Low Scissors	128
Seated Knee Tuck with Double Leg	125
Double Leg Raise with Low Range	123

SATURDAY – Rest Day

SUNDAY – Upper

Exercise	Page
Cobra	100
Reverse Dorsal Raise With Single Leg	107
Blackburn	105
Full Dorsal Raise with Fingers On Temples	100
Swimmer	112
Hand Push	66
Fast Hand Tap	74
W Formation	73
Pike Shoulder Press	77
Hand Grasp Pull	68
Straight Arm Chest Squeeze	89
Wide Hand Press Up	84
Plyo Press Up	91
Lateral Press Up	88
Front Loaded Press Up	87

WEEK 4 – UPPER BODY & LOWER BODY

MONDAY – Lower

Exercise	Page
Reverse Crunch	126
High Scissors	128
Shoulders Raised Lying Knee Tuck with Single Leg	124
Flutter Kick	126
Double Leg Raise	123
Heel Tap	135
Side Lying Oblique Crunch	134
Russian Twist with Bent Arms	136
Full Side Plank with Straight Arm	146
Forward Lunge	155
Wide Squat	157
Lateral Lunge	158
Side Lying Leg Lift with Forearm Resting	171
Kneeling Hydrant	163
Glute Bridge with Calf Raise	175

TUESDAY – Rest Day

WEDNESDAY – Upper

Exercise	Page
Close Hand Press Up	84
Lateral Press Up	88
Straight Arm Chest Squeeze	89
Plyo Press Up	91
Chest Squeeze	89
Superman	111
Dorsal Raise with Side Bend	103
Prone Heel Raise with Double Legs	108
Scapular Retraction with Bent Arms	115
Reverse Dorsal Raise with Double Leg	107
Hand Grasp Pull	68
T Formation	72
Fast Hand Tap	74
Pike Shoulder Press	77
Full Plank Bodysaw with Single Leg	75

THURSDAY – Lower

Exercise	Page
Squat with Rotation	152
Reverse Table Top	169
Down Dog with Leg Lift	161
Kneeling Leg Extension	162
Glute Bridge with Resting Bent Leg	166
Standing Calf Raise	172
Crunch with Raised Bent Knees	119
Plank	138
Seated Knee Tuck with Single Leg	125
Reverse Crunch	126
Opposite Vertical Toe Reach	121
Full Plank with Opposite Knee To Elbow	140
Oblique Crunch with Raised Bent Knees	133
Side Plank with Oblique Crunch	144
Bicycle Crunch	137

FRIDAY – Rest Day

SATURDAY – Upper

Exercise	Page
Y Formation	71
Fast Hand Tap	74
Full Plank Body Saw	75
Pike Shoulder Press	77
Side Single Arm Shoulder Wall Press	76
Wide Hand Press Up	84
Stacked Feet Press Up	86
Lateral Press up	88
Plyo Press Up	91
Plyo Staggered Hand Press Up	92
Blackburn	105
Dorsal Raise with Hands Clasped Behind Back	104
Swimmer	112
Prone Scissors	109
Full Dorsal Raise with Fingers On Temples	110

SUNDAY – Lower

Exercise	Page
Russian Twist with Bent Arms	136
Bicycle Crunch	137
Side Plank with Oblique Crunch	144
Full Side Plank with Straight Arm	146
Prisoner Squat	152
Diagonal Lunge	159
Lateral Lunge with Side Toe Touch	158
Reverse Lunge	156
Kneeling Step Up	161
Glute Bridge with Calf Raise Toe Tap	175
Crunch with Vertical Straight Legs	119
Reverse Crunch	126
Opposite Vertical Toe Reach	121
Hip Thrust	127
Seated Knee Tuck with Double Leg	125

WEEK 5 – PUSH, PULL & LEGS

MONDAY – Rest Day

TUESDAY – Pull

Exercise	Page
Down Dog Up Dog	101
Cat Cow	98
Fingertip Rotation	104
Full Dorsal Raise with Fingers On Temples	110
Scapular Retraction with Straight Arms	115
Crunch with Vertical Straight Legs	119
Reverse Crunch	126
Seated Knee Tuck with Double Leg	125
Flutter Kick	126
Hip Thrust	127
Oblique Crunch with Vertical Straight Legs	133
Heel Tap	135
Full Plank Sweep	140
Side Plank with Leg Lift	142
Full Side Plank with Leg Lift	147

WEDNESDAY – Legs

Exercise	Page
Prisoner Squat	152
Diagonal Lunge	159
Squat with Bent Knee Lift	153
Forward Lunge	155
Wall Sit with Bent Knee Lift	154
Kneeling Hydrant with Side Kick	165
Kneeling Bent Knee Heel Raise	163
Glute Bridge with Bent Knee Lift	167
Standing Calf Raise	172
Calf Raise with Single Leg	174

THURSDAY – Push

Exercise	Page
Stacked Feet Press Up	86
Staggered Hand Press Up	86
Front Loaded Press Up	87
Praying Hand Raise Chest Squeeze	90
Plyo Press Up	91
Plyo Staggered Hand Press Up	92
Hand Grasp Pull	68
Full Plank Body Saw	75
Y Formation	71
Side Single Arm Shoulder Wall Press	76
Pike Shoulder Press	77
Full Plank Body Saw with Single Leg	75

FRIDAY – Rest Day

SATURDAY – Pull

Exercise	Page
Side Lying Oblique Crunch	134
Bicycle Crunch	137
Russian Twist with Straight Arms	136
Side Plank with Leg Lift and Front Kick	143
Full Side Plank with Torso Rotation	147
Cobra	100
Cat Cow	98
Prone Scissors	109
Airplane	113
Back Pull	106
Reverse Crunch	126
Full Plank Body Saw with Single Leg	75
Hip Thrust	127
High Scissors	128
Plank	138

SUNDAY – Legs

Exercise	Page
Prisoner Squat	152
Reverse Lunge	156
Squat with Bent Knee Lift	153
Lateral Lunge with Side Toe Touch	158
Glute Bridge with High Straight Leg Lift	168
Kneeling Hydrant with Leg Extension	164
Reverse Table Top with Straight Leg Lift	169
Wall Sit	154
Glute Bridge with Calf Raise Toe Tap	175
Outward Calf Raise	173

WEEK 6 – PUSH, PULL & LEGS

MONDAY – Push

Exercise	Page
I Formation with Arms By Side	73
Standing Arm Drive	69
Fast Hand Tap	74
Full Plank Body Saw with Single Leg	75
T Formation	72
Pike Shoulder Press	77
Close Hand Press Up	84
Diamond Press Up	85
Straight Arm Chest Squeeze	89
Lateral Press Up	88
Plyo Staggered Hand Press Up	92
Single Arm Wall Press Up	81

TUESDAY – Pull

Exercise	Page
Vertical Toe Reach	120
Seated Knee Tuck with Double Leg	125
Low Scissors	128
Hip Thrust	127
Double Leg Raise	123
Oblique Crunch with Vertical Straight Legs	133
Russian Twist with Bent Arms	136
Full Plank Sweep	140
Full Side Plank with Leg Lift	147
Side Plank with Opposite Oblique Crunch	145
Fingertip Rotation	104
Reverse Dorsal Raise with Double Leg	107
Down Dog Up Dog	101
Dorsal Raise with Rotation	102
Swimmer	112

MONDAY – Rest Day

THURSDAY – Legs

Exercise	Page
Wide Squat	151
Lateral Lunge with Side Toe Touch	158
Diagonal Lunge	159
Glute Bridge with Low Straight Leg Lift	167
Falling Tower	160
Reverse Table Top	169
Kneeling Hydrant with Leg Extension	164
Seated Straight Leg Sweep	170
Glute Bridge with Calf Raise	175
Calf Raise with Single Leg	174

FRIDAY – Push

Exercise	Page
Wide Hand Press Up	84
Stacked Feet Press Up	86
Front Loaded Press Up	87
Plyo Press Up	91
Praying Hand Raise Chest Squeeze	90
Plyo Lateral Press Up	93
Fast Hand Tap	74
Full Plank Body Saw	75
T Formation	72
Pike Shoulder Press	77
Side Single Arm Shoulder Wall Press	76
Full Plank Body Saw with Single Leg	75

SATURDAY – Pull

Exercise	Page
Cobra	100
Prone Scissors	109
Down Dog Up Dog	101
Back Pull	106
Airplane	113
Crunch with Vertical Straight Legs	119
Vertical Toe Reach	120
Double Leg Raise	123
Full Plank Body Saw with Single Leg	75
Hip Thrust	127
Bicycle Crunch	137
Russian Twist with Straight Arms	136
Side Plank Leg Lift and Front Kick	143
Full Side Plank with Torso Rotation	147
Side Plank With Oblique Crunch	144

SUNDAY – Legs

Exercise	Page
Squat with Bent Knee Lift	153
Narrow Squat	151
Reverse Lunge	156
Lateral Lunge with Side Toe Touch	158
Glute Bridge with High Straight Leg Lift	168
Wall Sit with Bent Knee Lift	154
Kneeling Hydrant with Side Kick	165
Reverse Table Top with Straight Leg Lift	169
Glute Bridge with Calf Raise Toe Tap	175
Inward Calf Raise	173

WEEK 7 – CARDIO

MONDAY – Lactic Session

15 second run, 15 second recovery
30 second run, 30 second recovery
45 second run, 45 second recovery
60 second run, 60 second recovery
Intermediate: add on 90 second run, 90 second recovery
Advanced: add on 120 second run, 120 second recovery
Repeat the above routine 4 times. *Tip:* The aim is to stay at the same pace for each set.

TUESDAY – Rhythm Session

	Page
Beginner: 4 minute march **Intermediate:** 7 minute jog **Advanced:** 10 minute run	
Followed by:	
Jumping Jack x 3 sets	48
Power Knee Strike with Twist x 3 sets	45
Repeat the above routine 3 times. *Tip:* Rhythm sessions try to flush out the lactic from the previous days workout.	

WEDNESDAY – Tempo Session

30 second medium tempo pace
30 second jog
Continue for 5 minutes then 5 minute recovery
Repeat the above routine 5 times. *Tip:* The medium tempo pace is a speed that you are comfortable running at, but not a jog.

THURSDAY – Rhythm Session

	Page
Beginner: 4 minute march **Intermediate:** 7 minute jog **Advanced:** 10 minute run	
Followed by:	
Plyo Lateral Touch Down x 3 sets	59
Alternating Squat Thrust x 3 sets	46
Repeat the above routine 3 times.	

FRIDAY – Rest Day

SATURDAY – Speed Session

10 sets: 15 second sprint, 60 second recovery
Recovery time after 10 sets
Beginner: 5 minute recovery **Intermediate:** 4 minute recovery **Advanced:** 3 minute recovery
Repeat the above routine 3 times. *Tip:* Work as hard as you can on each interval, driving knees as high and fast as possible while simultaneously pumping your arms.

SUNDAY – Rhythm Session

	Page
Beginner: 7 minute march **Intermediate:** 10 minute jog **Advanced:** 15 minute run	
Followed by:	
Spotty Dog x 3 sets	53
Burpee x 3 sets	63
Repeat the above routine 3 times.	

WEEK 8 — CARDIO

MONDAY- Lactic Session

60 second run
30 second recovery
30 second run

Followed by 2 minute recovery

Beginner: 6 sets
Intermediate: 8 sets
Advanced: 10 sets

Tip: The aim here is to work hard on the 60 seconds, recover for 30 seconds and then run at tempo pace for the 30 seconds. This will flush out the lactic acid and make you ready for the next set after the 2 minute recovery.

TUESDAY — Rhythm Session

	Page
Beginner: 4 minute march **Intermediate:** 7 minute jog **Advanced:** 10 minute run	
Followed by:	
Squat Thrust x 3 sets	46
Plyo In Out Squat Jump x 3 sets	51
Repeat the above routine 3 times.	

Tip: Rhythm sessions try to flush out the lactic from the previous days workout.

WEDNESDAY — Tempo Session

60 second medium tempo pace
30 second jog
Continue for 6 minutes then 4 minute recovery

Repeat the above routine 4 times.

Tip: The 60 seconds should be your medium tempo pace and the 30 seconds should simply be light jogging.

THURSDAY — Rhythm Session

	Page
Beginner: 4 minute march **Intermediate:** 7 minute jog **Advanced:** 10 minute run	
Followed by:	
Plyo Power Skip x 3 sets	52
Burpee x 3 sets	63
Repeat the above routine 3 times.	

FRIDAY — Rest Day

SATURDAY — Speed Session

6 sets: 30 second sprint, 60 second recovery

Recovery time after 6 sets

Beginner: 5 minute recovery
Intermediate: 4 minute recovery
Advanced: 3 minute recovery

Repeat the above routine 2 times.

Tip: Work as hard as you can on each interval, driving knees as high and fast as possible while simultaneously pumping your arms.

SUNDAY — Rhythm Session

	Page
Beginner: 7 minute march **Intermediate:** 10 minute jog **Advanced:** 15 minute run	
Followed by:	
Plyo Lateral Bound x 3 sets	59
Plyo Lateral Squat Jump x 3 sets	58
Repeat the above routine 3 times.	

WEEK 9 – CARDIO

MONDAY – Lactic Session

Run (in seconds)	Recovery (in seconds)
Beginner	
30	30
45	45
60	60
90	90
120	120
90	90
60	60
45	45
30	30
Intermediate	
60	60
90	90
120	120
150	150
120	120
90	90
60	60
Advanced	
60	60
120	120
180	180
240	240
300	300
240	240
120	120
60	60

Tip: During this pyramid session, the aim is again to stay at a similar pace throughout the session and simply change the length of running time. The aim is to build up nicely to a 5 minute effort.

TUESDAY – Rhythm Session

	Page
Beginner: 5 minute march **Intermediate:** 8 minute jog **Advanced:** 12 minute run Followed by:	
Plyo Broad Jump x 3 sets	60
Tuck Jump x 3 sets	55
Repeat the above routine 3 times.	

Tip: Rhythm sessions try to flush out the lactic from the previous days workout.

THURSDAY – Rhythm Session

	Page
Beginner: 5 minute march **Intermediate:** 8 minute jog **Advanced:** 12 minute run Followed by:	
Plyo Diagonal Bound x 3 sets	61
Plyo Reverse Touchdown Power Skip x 3 sets	62
Repeat the above routine 3 times.	

SATURDAY – Speed Session

5 sets: 20 second sprint, 60 second recovery
5 sets: 10 second sprint, 45 second recovery
Recovery time after all 10 sets
Beginner: 5 minute recovery **Intermediate:** 4 minute recovery **Advanced:** 3 minute recovery
Repeat the above routine twice.

Tip: Work as hard as you can for each sprint, the different timings should give you different speed and lactic levels.

WEDNESDAY – Tempo Session

90 second medium tempo pace
30 second jog

Continue for 7 minutes then 3 minute recovery

Repeat the above routine 4 times.

Tip: Remember to stay controlled during this session with steady effort. The medium tempo pace is a speed that you are comfortable running at, but not a jog.

SUNDAY – Rhythm Session

	Page
Beginner: 8 minute march **Intermediate:** 12 minutes jog **Advanced:** 18 minute run Followed by:	
Plyo Sergeant Jump x 3 sets	57
Squat Thrust with Single Leg x 3 sets	47
Repeat the above routine 3 times.	

WEEK 10 – CARDIO

MONDAY – Lactic Session

15 second run, 15 second recovery
30 second run, 30 second recovery
45 second run, 45 second recovery
60 second run, 60 second recovery
Intermediate: add on 90 second run, 90 second recovery
Advanced: add on 120 second run, 120 second recovery
Repeat the above routine 5 times.

Tip: Aim to stay at the same pace for each set. You should see/feel an improvement from week 7, so judge how you feel and include extra sets or increase duration.

TUESDAY – Rhythm Session

	Page
Beginner: 8 minute march **Intermediate:** 12 minute jog **Advanced:** 18 minute run	
Followed by:	
Sumo Squat Thrust x 3 sets	47
Plyo Squat Jump x 3 sets	54
Repeat the above routine 3 times.	

Tip: Rhythm sessions try to flush out the lactic from the previous days workout.

WEDNESDAY – Tempo Session

120 second medium tempo pace 30 second jog
Continue for 8 minutes then 3 minute recovery
Repeat the above routine 4 times.

Tip: The medium tempo pace is a speed that you are comfortable running at, but not a jog.

THURSDAY – Rhythm Session

	Page
Beginner: 8 minute march **Intermediate:** 12 minute jog **Advanced:** 18 minute run	
Followed by:	
Burpee x 3 sets	63
Plyo Vertical Rocket Jump x 3 sets	55
Repeat the above routine 3 times.	

FRIDAY – Rest Day

SATURDAY – Speed Session

10 sets: 30 second sprint, 45 second recovery
Recovery time after 10 sets
Beginner: 5 minute recovery **Intermediate:** 4 minute recovery **Advanced:** 3 minute recovery
Repeat the above routine 3 times.

Tip: Work as hard as you can on each interval, driving knees as high and fast as possible while pumping your arms simultaneously.

SUNDAY – Rhythm Session

	Page
Beginner: 8 minute march **Intermediate:** 12 minute jog **Advanced:** 18 minute run	
Followed by:	
Plyo Reverse Touchdown Power Skip x 3 sets	62
Plyo Star Jump x 3 sets	56
Repeat the above routine 3 times.	

EXERCISE INDEX

ACKNOWLEDGEMENTS AND MY THANKS

My family and close friends, who came to visit, wrote to me and supported me in any way possible. I will always be grateful for your efforts and helping me along the way.

All inmates and anybody else using this book, who I hope will benefit and enjoy using it.

Pentonville staff and the Prison Service, who believed that I had a worthwhile idea and have made helped make this book available to inmates.

The Prince's Trust for their guidance and support.

All the people who have been involved in making this book a reality.

Lee Armstrong
Neil Barclay
Ingrid Bennett
James Cadwallader
Josh Cadwallader
Chris Christodoulou
Max Davies
Sam Dyer
Alanna Flanders
Ricky Flanders
Rachel Freeman
Joe Gelb

Mark Gray
Kate Hagger
Tony Hagger
Richard Hawkesworth
Oli Heeks
Richard Horsted
Gerry Hughes
Ieva Kazokaite
Bogdan Marius
Mum
Tom O'Donoghue

Andy Packer
Lee Pybus
Louisa Routledge
Toby Rowland
Drew Shearwood
Michael Smith
Dave Spence
Courtney Taylor
Terry Tew
Adrian Tribble
Andrew 'Shorty' Turner

CONTRIBUTORS

Drew Shearwood	Photography	www.drewshearwood.com
Josh Cadwallader	Logo Design	www.jrcad.co.uk
Toby Rowland	Technical Advice	www.tqrtraining.co.uk
Richard Horsted	Web Design	www.richardhorsted.com
Alanna Flanders	Makeup Artist	www.alannamua.com
3 Mills Studios	Film & TV Studios	www.3mills.com
Tony Hagger	Filming	www.a-zfilms.co.uk
Terry Tew	Sound & Lighting	www.terrytew.co.uk

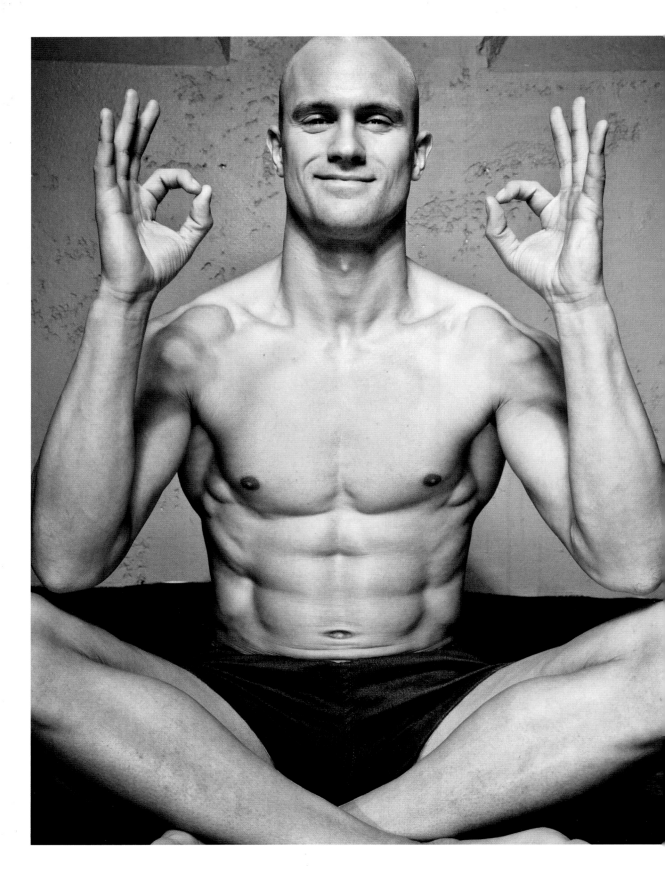